New —————
Health Tips
Encyclopedia

Edited by
Cal Beverly and
June Gunden

FC&A Publishing
103 Clover Green
Peachtree City, GA 30269

Printing and binding by Banta Company. Edited by Cal Beverly and June Gunden. Cover Design by Deberah Williams.

Tenth edition printed January 1992

ISBN 0-915099-20-9

Table of Contents

Introduction

The editors and publisher of this book have been diligent in attempting to provide accurate reproduction of the information contained in these newsletter articles. However, this book does not constitute medical advice and should not be construed as such. We cannot guarantee the safety or effectiveness of any drug or treatment or advice mentioned. The only intent of this book is to provide the consumer with easy-to-understand information. With the rapid advances in medicine and health care, we recommend in all cases that you contact your personal physician or health care provider before taking or discontinuing any medications, or before treating yourself in any way.

— The editors

viii

AGING

Longevity

Even though the average person in a developed country today lives to the age of 71, the life expectancy in 1900 was only 45. Many, of course, live longer than the average, and while at present the 85th year seems to be a sort of "barrier," there is reason to hope that one day most of us will survive in good health to 115 (the full potential life span), the *New England Journal of Medicine* (312:1159) reports.

Research with various animal species all points to the same conclusion — that life is longest when the food supply is limited sufficiently to keep the body weight just below average. Furthermore, all natural and artificial substances that extend animals' lives, in addition, cause some limitation of weight. Possibly, therefore, it is the ability of exercise and substances such as Gerovital, Levodopa, and Superioxide Dismutase to limit weight rather than anything else that allows them to be effective in delaying aging and prolonging life. The Rumanian makers of Gerovital have advertised that this substance is effective against aging, and, indeed, it has increased the life span of rodents. Studies in humans, however, have not shown a significant anti-aging effect. Neither do we have any convincing evidence that vitamins A, C, or E in large doses have anti-aging effects, nor even that they are safe. Actually, in one study, high vitamin E doses increased mortality. So, while we wait for the answer to aging, we should try to stay lean and avoid consumption of anything dangerous like tobacco, even though it helps to keep us slim.

Anti-Aging Cosmetics

Cosmetic companies are claiming that some of their products can rejuvenate the skin by working at a "cellular" level, implying that the ingredients penetrate the skin deeply before they get down to work. Most such products are very expensive and contain, among other things, trace quantities of collagen or some of the body's natural hormones.

If these creams really did any good, *Cutis* (39:23) points out, they would need to be classified as prescription drugs (like Retin-A), and claims that the ingredients have rejuvenating effects are akin to suggesting that blood transfusions can be given by rubbing blood on the skin. Such claims are "pure puffery," according to a recent article in *Time* magazine.

Some of the "natural" substances in these "skin renewal," "wrinkle-removing," "rejuvenating," and "sun damage-repairing" formulas have also caused allergic skin reactions, so don't expect them to be better than any other skin creams. About the only good these expensive cosmetics can do is to moisturize the skin and thereby to make it appear a little more smooth. However, the much less expensive skin moisturizing products will do exactly the same thing. Keeping your skin moist (which means keeping the air indoors moist as well) and shielding it from the sun will, more than anything, help to keep your skin's appearance young.

Unrecognized Pneumonia, a Threat to the Elderly

Whereas pneumonia in children and younger adults tends to be an easily recognized illness with abrupt onset, flushing of the skin, fever, cough, shortness of breath, and pain in the chest on breathing, the same infection in older people causes so many fewer and less dramatic symptoms that the disease may be easily overlooked, *Emergency Medicine* (18#1:52) reports.

In the elderly, therefore, pneumonia is often left undiagnosed and untreated until it is too late, and is a common cause of death. Even when the doctor examines an older person who has pneumonia, he may not find any typical signs during the first few days of the illness. Often, the only abnormalities may be slight fever, lack of desire for food and drink, signs of dehydration (such as dryness of the mouth, hollow cheeks, sunken eyes, and little if any urination) with mental slowness and loss of alertness.

Older people with these clues of illness, therefore, should be taken to the hospital without delay so that X-rays and blood tests can be performed to establish the diagnosis, and so that treatment can be started without delay. In some cases, however, the doctor may not wish to move the patient. Instead, he will make a tentative diagnosis of pneumonia without X-rays or tests and start treatment at home with an antibiotic, such as penicillin, right away.

If treated in time, most cases begin to respond within 24 hours and thereafter gradually improve until they have become normal again after several days. Complications and slower responses are common, however, when treatment is delayed, if there is an underlying illness (such as heart failure), or in the very old. Since pneumonia is so common, so easily overlooked, and so potentially dangerous, we must all be alert to this possibility, even when an elderly person appears to be just vaguely unwell.

Memory and Medicines

Certain medications, the *American Family Physician* (32#2:250) reports, interfere with our ability to store information in our memories and quickly recall it on demand. Older people, many of whom already have this problem, tend to be much more severely affected.

The drugs in question share a common mechanism of action—they block production of a substance known as acetyl choline in the tissues. Acetyl choline is responsible for many functions in the body, including memory functions of the brain. Since production of this substance naturally declines in many older people to the extent that the memory becomes impaired, drugs that interfere with acetyl choline production tend to make an older person's memory very much worse. The drugs that do this include many medications used for insomnia, for calming the nerves, for reducing tremors, or for decreasing the production of gastric acid.

Since saliva and mucus secretion also depend upon acetyl choline's presence in the tissues, all of these drugs additionally produce dryness of the mouth. Whenever possible, therefore, older people with memory problems should try to do without any drug that causes dryness.

Dehydration: Special Danger for the Elderly

As we grow older, we gradually lose our sense of thirst and can become dangerously dehydrated without realizing it. The *New England Journal of Medicine* (311,753) reports that elderly people tend not to drink enough to make up for the fluids lost by excessive sweating during infections or fever or following treatment with a diuretic ("water pill").

In a study at Oxford, a group of men 67 to 75 years old was compared with another group aged 20 to 31. After 24 hours without fluids, the older men experienced surprisingly little thirst or discomfort, whereas the younger men were anxious to drink copious amounts of fluid. The older men were just as dehydrated as the younger ones but did not take as much of the fluid made freely available to everybody. Even though we do not know the cause of this difference in behavior, it is important to recognize it and to make up for it as we grow older by routinely drinking several glasses of water every day.

Like all other creatures, we are composed mainly of water. Soon after conception, the embryo is about 90 percent water but changes throughout gestation, so that just before birth the fetus is only about 80 percent water. By the time we reach maturity the percentage is 70 percent, and in our old age it falls below 60 percent, *Geriatrics* (42#6:53) reports. Since water is a good insulator, as we grow older we have trouble keeping warm during cold weather and staying cool when it is hot.

Making life still more difficult for senior citizens, old kidneys are less able than young ones to produce concentrated urine. Therefore, complications of dehydration in the elderly include kidney diseases (infections and stones) and excessive responses to medications that are eliminated from the body through the kidneys. Drugs affected by this include many hypertension drugs, heart medicines, and "water pills."

Most seriously, what would be only a minor ailment in a young person could be the final illness for someone older who is dehydrated, *Drug Therapy* (17#1:56) reports. Elderly persons who become dehydrated have a much higher than expected mortality rate from infections because, when they do not drink enough to make up for their fluid losses (from sweating and vomiting, etc.), their blood becomes so much thicker that their kidneys cannot filter it well enough to get rid of body wastes. A vicious cycle occurs when consciousness becomes impaired by these wastes accumulating in the blood. The victim is then no longer able to drink extra fluid even when advised to do so. Administration of fluids intravenously becomes necessary.

To avoid these potentially very serious problems, older people must realize that thirst is no longer a reliable guide to their fluid needs, but often lags two to three days behind actual requirements. When healthy, a simple rule of thumb is to drink enough fluids to keep the urine a pale yellow rather than dark in color and to keep it coming in fair volume (at least four pints of urine daily). When you are ill or have fever, you should make it a point to drink more than usual, unless told otherwise.

A good way to make sure that you do not become dehydrated when taking exercise in a hot climate is to weigh yourself several times a day and to drink a pint of fluid for every pound that you have lost. Since prevention is better than cure, you should also drink one to two pints of fluid half an hour before taking part in any prolonged types of exercise, such as a few sets of tennis or 18 holes of golf.

Heat Stroke in the Elderly

During hot weather, heat stroke fatalities occur 12-15 times more often in the elderly than in younger people, the *U.S. Pharmacist* (9#6:23) reports. The elderly are more prone to heat stroke because they cannot very easily get rid of their excess body heat by sweating.

For body heat to evaporate, enough blood must circulate through the skin to support extra sweating. If the heart cannot easily pump that much blood, or if the blood volume has become depleted by dehydration, insufficient blood reaches the sweat glands. As pointed out in the previous section, dehydration is commonly caused by a diuretic ("water pill") drug that is being taken by people with heart failure or hypertension to increase the urine output. Several other drugs, including some stomach medicines and antihistamines, have a skin-drying effect that may also interfere with sweating.

So, in very hot weather, even if they are feeling well, older people should spend more time in air-conditioned places and avoid sitting in direct sunlight, particularly if they are taking any medication. If exposure to heat is unavoidable, they should try to compensate by drinking more, and (since exertion generates heat) by becoming much less physically active. *Geriatrics* (41#5:108) recommends that when older people begin an exercise program in warm weather or after traveling to a warmer climate, they should limit the intensity and duration of the exercise at first and only gradually increase it over a period of 10 to 14 days.

Laxative Overuse

Thirty percent of people older than 60 take laxatives regularly and about three percent overuse them dangerously, *Geriatrics* (40#10:5) reports. Overuse of laxatives is like a drug addiction in that the body becomes dependent upon them, as it is alternately overstimulated, then abnormally quieted.

This latter phase is often accompanied by an uncomfortable sensation of being bloated, which encourages the person to take another dose of laxative just at the time when it is not needed. Drastically overstimulated in this way, the intestine wall leaks excessive amounts of body fluid, which are elimi-nated as watery stools. Evacuated with the stools are vital minerals, which are not easily replaced in older persons. One such mineral is calcium (see the next section), which is particularly harmful since osteoporosis from loss of bone calcium is already a problem for the elderly.

Accordingly, we should regulate our bowels by dietary means alone, using fluid, salad, fruit, bran, etc., or we are likely to have trouble with our bones in old age.

Absorbing Calcium

If one takes a dietary supplement of calcium, it will not do any good unless there is acid in the stomach to dissolve it and prepare it for absorption, the *American Family Physician* (34#3:188) reports. This is one reason why older people lack calcium and develop brittle bones: they cannot absorb enough calcium to keep their bones strong when their stomachs can no longer secrete enough acid.

To maximize calcium absorption, older people should take their tablets of calcium with meals because when the stomach is filled with food, it produces more acid than at any other time

Nosebleeds in the Elderly

Nosebleeds, infrequent during most of our adult lives, again become more common after 70. Whereas nasal hemor-rhages in children are mostly due to trauma (nosepicking, etc.) and are usually easy to stop, nosebleeds in the elderly usually reflect some more general disturbance and can result in a heavy blood loss. Perhaps the most common cause for nasal bleeding in the elderly is the combined effect of brittle, hardened arteries and high blood pressure. Although, in most cases, simply squeezing the nose for five minutes usually stops the bleeding, medication to control the blood pressure and cauterization of the bleeding nasal artery are also often needed to prevent recurrences.

Now, according to the *British Medical Journal,* we should be on the lookout for two additional factors in the elderly. Many elderly people have such poor diets that they become borderline cases of scurvy (vitamin C deficiency resulting in hemorrhages). This can be quickly corrected with ascorbic acid (vitamin C) tablets, one gram daily. Another common factor is the long-continued use of anti-arthritic drugs. Aspirin and most anti-arthritis drugs (with names ending in "-profen") slow blood clotting and therefore help to cause bleeding. When this is so, treatment with aspirin, etc., may need to be temporarily discontinued and later taken at a lower dose. In some cases, it may be necessary to avoid these drugs entirely.

Dizziness from Aspirin

Sudden spells of dizziness, possibly leading to falls, become an increasing problem as we age, *Geriatrics* (41#7:31) reports. In some cases, the dizziness is a symptom of serious disorders, such as abnormal heart rhythms or "little strokes," which need to be treated before they get any worse. Accordingly, anyone developing mysterious dizzy spells should tell a doctor about them right away.

Fortunately, however, dizziness is often not due to anything serious. In fact, many cases occur as a result of taking certain medicines, including aspirin, and clear up after they have been discontinued. Not all medications, however, have such reversible effects, and several (such as the antibiotics gentamicin or streptomycin) often cause dizziness followed by permanent hearing loss.

Because aspirin is usually taken without a doctor's orders and is often not regarded as a "drug," it is frequently overlooked as the cause of repeated dizzy spells.

Vitamin D Needs of the Elderly

To make sure that our bones remain strong and are not too easily fractured in old age, it is essential that we get not only sufficient calcium (1.5-2 grams every day) but also enough vitamin D. Since vitamin D is responsible for efficient absorption of calcium from the diet and for calcium's retention by the bones, lack of this vitamin is now regarded as an often overlooked factor in the loss of calcium and the fractures that occur in so many older adults.

A poor dietary intake is not the only cause of vitamin D deficiency, *Geriatrics* (40#8:45) reports. Other causes include chronic diarrhea, gall bladder disease, kidney failure, absence of the stomach (after its removal because of an ulcer or cancer), alcoholism, liver disease, and certain medications (anticonvulsants and some cholesterol-lowering drugs).

Another factor, *Geriatrics* (42#7:30) reports, is that old skin is less efficient than young skin at producing vitamin D when exposed to the ultraviolet light in sunshine. Adults, in addition, are becoming increasingly concerned (and rightfully so) about skin cancer, which is likely to occur if the skin is exposed excessively to the sun. However, while minimizing exposure of our skin to the sun, we must take care as we grow older to avoid letting ourselves become deficient of vitamin D.

Normally, we need to get at least 400 units of vitamin D

every day and may need twice that much if there is any doubt about our ability to absorb it. However, adults are less likely than children to take vitamin supplements (many older people try to save money by not buying them).

To avoid a vitamin D deficiency, *Geriatrics* recommends, elderly persons should be exposed outdoors to sunshine at least 15 minutes twice a week. When this is not possible, it is essential that they be given a supplement of the vitamin by mouth.

Vitamin C

When an older person complains of swollen lower legs, heart failure is usually to blame. However, another cause that is often overlooked is scurvy, a disease due to lack of vitamin C.

Elderly men who live alone and do their own cooking are especially prone to a deficiency of this vitamin because they tend not to eat enough fruits and vegetables. Even if they eat out from time to time, they tend not to choose the right foods, the *Journal of the American Medical Association* (253:805) reports.

Scurvy is a likely diagnosis if, in addition to swelling of the legs, there is painful stiffness of the knees and ankles, and if there is a bumpy rash with tiny hemorrhages around each hair follicle. This diagnosis is easily confirmed by measuring the blood level of vitamin C.

Treatment, which should be given by a doctor, involves correcting the deficiency and then improving the diet. Food faddists and those who avoid acid foods (such as oranges) because of an ulcer or indigestion are also prime candidates for deficiency of vitamin C.

Teeth and Aging

Loss of teeth used to be thought of as a natural part of aging, but now, according to *Postgraduate Medicine* (75#5:231), this is open to question. It is believed that many older people lose teeth because they have poor diets, lack vitamins, or have dental disease. Among the tooth-destroying afflictions of the elderly, xerostomia (dryness of the mouth) is perhaps the most common.

Saliva, apparently, has an anti-bacterial effect that protects teeth, and anything that reduces the salivary flow hastens dental decay. Decreased saliva secretion is not a function of aging per se but, rather, is a side effect of many drugs that older people take. Drugs most responsible for doing this are the anti-cholinergics (those used to decrease gastric acid secretion and relieve pain in the stomach).

Others causing xerostomia include the antidepressants, antihistamines, antihypertensives, anticancer drugs, decongestants, tranquilizers, and diuretics ("water pills"). If it is not possible to do without these drugs or to reduce their dosage, a salivary substitute spray, such as Xero-Lube or Salivart, should be employed as often as necessary to keep the mouth comfortably moist.

Indigestion after 40

Most people with episodes of discomfort or pain in the middle of the upper abdomen assume that they must have indigestion, whereas with the same sort of pain in the lower chest they are more likely to suspect heart trouble.

For young people, this diagnosing by the location of pain is usually reliable, but as people grow older it becomes increasingly misleading. In fact, the *Postgraduate Medical Journal* (60:338) points out that anyone over 40 who repeatedly complains of indigestion pains for the first time in his life should be assumed to have heart disease instead. It is only safe to assume that the pain is truly due to a disorder of the stomach in such cases when heart trouble has been ruled out by negative blood tests and a normal ECG (heart tracing).

Water Pill (Diuretic) Danger in the Elderly

Many elderly people take medication regularly every day that helps them to eliminate salt and water from the tissues. Usually, this is started as part of the treatment for high blood pressure or heart disease.

However, if continued indefinitely and without tests being performed to determine whether it is still necessary, the medication can reduce the salt and water in the body to levels which are extremely low, the *Archives of Internal Medicine* (146:1295) reports. Unfortunately, the changes usually take place so gradually that this condition is often overlooked until the patient has slid into a coma and begun to convulse.

Warning signs that too much salt and water have been lost include weakness, drowsiness, slow thinking, and mental withdrawal, all of which can be too easily attributed to the person's advancing age. Perhaps, in some cases, what seems to be the behavior of senile dementia (Alzheimer's disease) may actually be due to a lack of salt. The victims, furthermore, are usually elderly women of well below average body weight, whose health appears, at the best of times, to be somewhat delicate.

If this condition is caught early enough and before the patient has experienced unconsciousness and convulsions, treatment by discontinuing the diuretic drug and giving some extra salt and potassium (in the form of fruit juice) is usually rapidly successful. More severe cases must be taken to the hospital without delay for treatment with special intravenous fluids.

To avoid this type of problem, older people must not take a diuretic medicine indefinitely without seeing a doctor, especially if they are already on a low salt diet and are not eating and drinking well.

Cool Surroundings Dangerous for the Elderly

An expert on aging, according to the *Journal of the American Medical Association* (243:47), believes that the risk of death from hypothermia (body coldness) in the elderly has been greatly underestimated. The expert believes that many elderly people with heart disease or pneumonia really die from the effects of low body temperature rather than from the illnesses listed in their death certificates.

Elderly people do not always sense how cold they are, and this, combined with a decline in the ability of their bodies to conserve and generate heat when needed, makes it difficult for them to tolerate cool surroundings. Even when they are not ill, and the room temperature does not fall below 65° F (18°C), older people can slide slowly, over a period of several days, into a dangerous state of hypothermia.

Nowadays, as we try to conserve energy during the winter by keeping our houses cooler, electric blankets and long underwear become essential for older members of the family.

AIDS

AIDS Virus in Saliva

Free AIDS virus is much more plentiful in the saliva of infected persons than it is in their genital secretions, letters to the editor of the *British Medical Journal* (294:705) assert. AIDS virus, therefore, is more likely to be transmitted from person to person during open-mouth kissing than by sexual intercourse, the correspondents believe. The fact that kissing and intercourse usually occur at the same time has probably led to the erroneous assumption that semen and vaginal secretions are the most potent sources of the AIDS virus, they suggest.

If this is true, condoms are unlikely to provide much help in preventing AIDS virus infection. Whether saliva is really so important a source of AIDS virus will need to be confirmed with careful laboratory studies. Nevertheless, the dental profession has long been concerned and takes precautions to minimize the risk of infection from saliva. Everyone, of course, should be alert to the fact that even "healthy" people who have become infected with the virus, but who have not yet developed any signs or symptoms of AIDS, can easily pass the virus on to others.

Some people have become indignant about the report that saliva of persons infected with the AIDS virus might be infectious. The "party line" on AIDS still seems to be that only members of the high risk groups need be greatly concerned about this epidemic killer disease. The rest of us, many feel, can safely carry on as usual.

In the interest of fair balance, we are therefore reporting a case of AIDS that, according to a letter to the editor of the *New England Journal of Medicine* (318:1203), was conveyed from husband to wife solely by kissing.

The husband acquired AIDS from blood transfusions he had received during major surgery, an operation that rendered him permanently impotent. After the operation, kissing his wife was his only sexual activity. Salivary transmission thus seems to have been responsible for the spread of AIDS from this man to his wife.

Predictably, of course, some of the "experts" suggested that we have no proof that the wife remained faithful to her husband, and that, therefore, her AIDS should not be cited as proving the possibility of salivary transmission.

Since AIDS is a killer disease, and because the dental profession is concerned enough about the salivary transmission of the AIDS virus that they wear rubber gloves, why should we all not be equally concerned? Also, why do the authorities now recommend using a tube for mouth-to-mouth resuscitation?

The chances of acquiring AIDS by kissing a stranger may be very small, we agree, but is it wise to deny that there is at least some risk? Even the National Institute of Dental Research talks about a "low risk," not a zero risk, in its report on an anti-AIDS substance in saliva in the *Journal of the American Dental Association* (116:635).

AIDS and Zinc

A recent edition of the *Journal of the American Medical Association (JAMA)* (259:817,839) contains information about two aspects of AIDS.

The first was the summary of an article that had appeared in the famous English scientific journal, *Nature*, reporting how long it takes after a blood transfusion containing the AIDS virus before recipients come down with the disease. This depends on age, it was found. Children have the shortest incubation period, just under two years, while with adults it is about six to eight years.

The second story appeared in a letter to the editor of *JAMA* from some scientists in Italy who found that the depressed immunity of AIDS is associated with depressed blood levels of zinc and of a hormone from the thymus, a gland that is involved in controlling the body's defenses against infection of all kinds.

Furthermore, they discovered, the depressed thymus hormone levels in the blood of AIDS patients can instantly be restored to normal by the addition of some zinc.

On the basis of these observations, which were all made on blood samples in the laboratory, they speculate that giving zinc to AIDS patients might well help to boost their immunity against infections and, thereby, ward off those fatal infections to which all AIDS victims ultimately succumb. At the very least, this seems worth trying and, no doubt, will be the subject of further research.

AIDS Virus in Swimming Pools

The prevailing attitude toward the spread of AIDS is that the causative virus for this fatal disease is spread by sexual intercourse, the injection of blood or products derived from it, or by sharing contaminated needles or syringes. Most people feel there is no evidence of spread by ordinary social contact, such as the sharing of washing facilities, eating utensils, or toilet facilities, etc.

One possible exception to the rule that "ordinary social contact" is always safe, an editorial in the *British Medical Journal* (293:221) reports, is the sharing of swimming pools and whirlpools with persons harboring AIDS virus. Although the editorial bows to convention in using the words "extremely unlikely" when discussing the possibility that the AIDS virus could be spread in this way, it does nevertheless go so far as to suggest that it might be under certain circumstances, such as if a lot of people share a public bathing facility, or if there is not enough disinfectant in the water to kill the virus quickly.

The editorial suggests that the danger of acquiring AIDS virus from contaminated swimming pools would be greater if one had a recent laceration (cut) or abrasion (scraped area) of the skin through which virus particles could gain entry to the tissues. Also, it was suggested, since viruses get into the body more easily through mucous membranes than through the skin, swallowing large amounts of water (as some small children do) conceivably could be dangerous.

Although it has never been proved that AIDS virus can be spread in swimming pools, the *Journal* editorial does suggest that, at least theoretically, this is possible. "Heresy" though this may be, it is the thinking of a very learned man, Professor Arie Zuckerman, chairman of Microbiology of London's School of Hygiene and Tropical Medicine.

AIDS and Psoriasis

The sudden development of psoriasis in an adult who has not had it before and who has no family history of psoriasis, especially if it is unusually severe, should make one suspect that the victim is also infected with the AIDS virus, *Cutis* (39:347) reports.

Psoriasis, it will be recalled, is a chronic dermatitis with raised patches of red, scaly skin that itch severely. It is not ordinarily infectious, but in people who have AIDS as well, there may be weeping skin lesions that shed the AIDS virus. In AIDS victims, furthermore, psoriasis tends to be more extensive, severe, treatment-resistant, and even life-threatening. One is reluctant to give these patients steroids (cortisone-like drugs) since they depress immunity, and AIDS victims already have difficulty in resisting infections.

AIDS patients with weeping lesions with psoriasis become extremely vulnerable to bacterial infections. Accordingly, for both parties concerned, it would be much safer to avoid any physical contact.

The AIDS "Breakout"

While New York City has 29 percent of all AIDS victims in the United States (San Francisco 10 percent, Los Angeles 9 percent, Miami 3 percent, Newark 2 percent), the remaining 47 percent of people with AIDS live in smaller communities throughout the country. *Modern Medicine* (55#10:80) reports that one recently diagnosed patient is a farmer who milks 40 cows every morning and evening.

For every person with AIDS, there are about 100 others who do not yet have the disease, but who have become infected with the virus. Most of these people will ultimately develop AIDS and die from it sometime during the next three to 10 years, authorities believe.

Despite this chilling evidence of spread, many commentators who lack the necessary information and understanding have been suggesting that the worst is over, and that AIDS remains essentially a disease of homosexuals, drug addicts, and members of certain urban minority groups, among whom it has already peaked. This is not only untrue, but it lulls people into a false sense of security and suggests that we need no longer take steps to defend ourselves against this killer disease.

Returning to plain facts, the virus has already infected 11 percent of prostitutes nationwide, is showing up more and more often in our "normal" heterosexual population, and public health authorities are now talking about the start of "the breakout" phase in the spread of AIDS throughout the U.S.A. Casual sex coupled with ignorance of the facts about the epidemic provide nearly ideal conditions for the spread of this disease. Furthermore, so long as our TV personalities, movies, magazines, and commercials continue presenting sex as an attractive recreational activity, many people will have difficulty in viewing it otherwise and in seeing the need for safer behavior.

If we are to halt the transmission of AIDS, the Surgeon General believes we must do a better job in educating people about it and in getting them to become more responsible in their relationships with one another.

ALLERGIES

Recognizing Drug Allergies

Since one in 20 hospital admissions results from an

allergic drug reaction, yours could easily be one of them. Recognizing the symptoms of drug allergy and taking prompt action could help you to avoid serious complications. Allergic reactions to drugs occur when the drug or its "breakdown" product combine with a body protein and "turn on" the immune system (cells and organs your body uses to fight illness).

According to the book *Immunologic Diseases* (1:413, Little Brown & Co.), allergic reactions can be immediate — occurring within minutes of taking the drug; or they may be delayed — occurring up to several days after you finish your course of drug therapy. Fever, lymph node swelling, joint pain, asthma, runny nose, hives, or (most common) rashes may all indicate drug allergy. Sensitivity to sunlight may also be caused by your body's altered response to a drug.

If you suspect that you're allergic to something that your doctor has prescribed, stop taking it immediately, and call him for instructions. Severe symptoms may be treated with other drugs, but most will disappear after you stop taking the medicine. If you are allergic to any drug, be sure not to take it again, because those who initially have a mild reaction may have a much more profound (even fatal) one the next time.

Allergic Noses

To identify the triggering substance responsible for allergic nasal symptoms (such as stuffiness, itching, redness, and watering), it is most helpful to ask about both the season and the times of day when attacks occur.

Thus, *Emergency Medicine* (16#10:20) reports, summertime attacks that begin about mid-morning are probably due to pollen and do not occur earlier in the day because the morning dew dampens the pollen dust and keeps it out of the air. Attacks that occur indoors year round are more likely due to house dust or pet dander. Mold sensitivity is at its worst during damp, rainy weather, but attacks can be triggered by air blown into the face from a car's air conditioner or room humidifier (both offer dark, damp, favorable habitats for mold growth).

The best treatment is to avoid exposure to the trigger substance and to reduce its concentration in one's surroundings as much as possible. In the case of molds, this involves drying up damp basements, etc., changing filters, cleaning humidifiers regularly, spraying with Lysol, and keeping closets dry with a constantly lit bulb. Getting mold out of a car's air conditioner can be difficult and usually requires a mechanic's help.

When measures such as these fail to provide relief, help can be obtained from antihistamine pills and, if necessary, desensitization shots as well. Antihistamines work best when they are taken around the clock to prevent allergic attacks and are not so effective when begun after an attack has already occurred. A common mistake is to take an antihistamine, get better, and then stop taking it. For more difficult cases, the allergist may need to prescribe other drugs in addition.

One type of allergy that has often been overlooked, the *American Family Physician* (29#5:408) reports, is triggered by grass pollen and is usually brought on by mowing the lawn. In the past, this allergy has generally been assumed to be caused by the leaves (blades) of grass, weeds, or the molds deposited on them, but, understandably, it has not been too responsive to desensitization shots aimed specifically at those causes.

Water Pills and Sunlight

Certain drugs have the ability to induce an allergic hypersensitivity to sunlight, a side effect known as phototoxicity. Perhaps the most common medicines to do this are the thiazide diuretics ("water pills") that so many people rely upon for the control of high blood pressure or heart failure.

Phototoxic effects in the skin include itching and a red, bumpy rash (due to many small blisters) on parts of the body exposed to sunlight. When the drug is stopped right away, the rash may quickly disappear, even if it continues to be exposed to the sun. However, if the drug is ever given again, the rash quickly returns and will continue to cause discomfort for the rest of the person's life whenever he or she is exposed to sunlight.

In such cases, it may be possible to shield the skin with PUVA (an artificial deep suntan). To do this, the *Archives of Dermatology* (121:522) reports, dermatologists give an artificial vitamin A-like drug by mouth that, after it is absorbed, darkens the skin in the presence of ultraviolet light (UV), while they administer graded doses of UV. Without such treatment, people who have chronic phototoxicity must permanently avoid the sun.

Chewing Gum Allergy

Not usually thought of as something to which one might become allergic, chewing gum does sometimes cause reactions of this kind, a writer to the editor of the *Lancet* (1:617) points out. His letter reports the case of a woman who developed a skin reaction due to an allergic type of inflammation of her blood vessels.

After many tests, it was found that she was reacting to butylated hydroxytoluene (BHT), the antioxidant preservative that is added to many foods such as cake mixes, potato chips, salted peanuts, dehydrated mashed potatoes, and some chewing gums. The lady's skin began clearing four days after she stopped chewing gum but flared up again a few hours after a test dose of BHT. So, if you use chewing gum and develop an unexplained allergy or skin disease, it is possible that you are reacting to BHT.

Humidifier Fever

Like Legionnaire's Disease, this illness can be conveyed in ventilating systems. Termed "Monday Sickness," outbreaks occur only in buildings supplied with humidified air.

The few affected people, according to reports in the *British Medical Journal* and the *New England Journal of Medicine*, are those who become allergic to particles carried in moisture droplets. The particles are fragments of dead microorganisms and fungi that were living in damp recesses of the humidification system. People who react to them typically begin having problems four to six weeks after starting work in the affected environment.

During the evening of the first day back at work each week, they have slight fever, shivering, headache, aching muscles, and a tight feeling in the chest. By next day, they are usually well again except for a mild cough with small amounts of white sputum. Nothing is found on examination of these people except evidence in their blood of hypersensitivity to the offending organisms. This illness is not serious, poses no permanent threat to the health, and can be eliminated by regularly cleansing the humidifier.

Home Humidifiers

When the house is heated and sealed against the cold outside, the warm, dry air indoors picks up water from wherever it can, including the mucous membranes of your nose, throat, and lungs. In yielding moisture to the air, your respiratory passages become dried out, and this can set the stage for repeated attacks of croup, nosebleeds, and middle ear infections in small children, and for sinusitis, chronic bronchitis, and asthma in people of any age. By adding water to the air of your home with a vaporizer or humidifier, you can do a lot to eliminate these problems.

Reviewing the various appliances that are on the market for this purpose, the *U.S. Pharmacist* (7#11:35) clearly favors humidifiers (which produce water droplets) over vaporizers (that produce mist or steam). The latter tend to use more energy, are more likely to cause burns and scalds, and require more attention to be kept working. While both kinds of appliance may harbor molds and bacteria that can be spread with water particles throughout the house, humidifiers are the more likely to become contaminated.

Allergies and infections have been reported in connection with the micro-organisms in humidifiers, but by far the most noticeable problem associated with them is their offensive odor. To prevent this, the *U.S. Pharmacist* reports, one should add a quarter of a cupful of household chlorine bleach to an appliance that has been nearly filled with water. Because chlorine fumes are hazardous, this procedure should be performed out of doors. After running the appliance with the diluted bleach solution for about one and a half hours, it should be drained and rinsed a couple of times with fresh water before being brought in and returned to use. Repeat this procedure every few weeks to keep your humidifier clean and odor-free. This is more efficient than trying to stop contamination by adding disinfectants or other chemicals to the water. They may smell nice, but they can be quite irritating to the respiratory passages and thereby do more harm than they prevent. None of this applies to the newest humidifiers that work ultrasonically. They, nevertheless, need to be occasionally cleaned.

Herbal Tea

Herbal teas are fashionable these days, and many people regard them as a refreshing caffeine-free alternative to coffee and ordinary tea. Many even believe that they must have beneficial effects because they are sold in health food stores.

Actually, according to *Emergency Medicine* (18#20:21), many herbal teas are potentially much less safe than conventional tea and are capable of producing headaches, diarrhea, dermatitis, asthma, insomnia, heart rhythm disturbances, seizures, and liver disease (even cancer) when taken regularly for a long time.

It may be difficult to recognize these dangers since the side effects usually do not begin until one has taken the herbal product for several weeks. Thus, when trouble does appear, one is unlikely to make the association and may continue drinking the tea. Furthermore, since herbal products are considered to be neither foods nor drugs, they are not under the Food and Drug Administration's control.

So, just because they are sold by your supermarket and health food store, you cannot assume that herbal teas are safe. Chamomile, comfrey, ginseng, gordolobo yerba, and impila are among the herbal products reported to do harm sometimes.

Since chamomile is cross-allergenic with aster, chrysanthe-
mum, and ragweed, when an allergic individual drinks a cup
of chamomile tea he may experience asthma, hay fever, or
hives.

ALZHEIMER'S DISEASE

Aluminum and Alzheimer's Disease

Alzheimer's disease (once called senile dementia), is a
dreaded condition that afflicts about one in three people in
their 80s. The gradual accumulation of aluminum in the brain
over a lifetime has been thought by many experts to be a
contributory cause to the disease, if not the main one.

That view has not been universal, however. Other experts
have argued that there is no relationship between the amount
of aluminum in the brain and the degree of the dementia. Their
objection is now weakened by research reported in the *Lancet*
(1:354) that used the newest and most refined method (nuclear
magnetic resonance) for studying the chemistry of the brain.

The research consistently showed a minute deposit of
aluminum in the very center of each and every nerve cell
"tangle," the characteristic lesion of the brain in all cases of
Alzheimer's. This presence of aluminum at the center of every
tangle strongly suggests that it is involved in the initiation of
the Alzheimer's patient's brain damage.

Though some experts believe that the aluminum found in
these brain lesions has merely settled out of the blood stream
into tissues that already have been damaged by something

else, there is evidence that points to the contrary. It has been shown that aluminum inhibits the enzyme in our tissues (called choline esterase) that is known to be responsible for maintaining normal functioning of the brain. Thus, far from being merely a "passive marker" that settles out of the blood into damaged parts of the brain, aluminum could be the cause of the damage as well.

Furthermore, there is current news of a dementia that is similar to that of Alzheimer's, but accelerated, that has been occurring in kidney failure patients undergoing dialysis when the dialysis fluid is made from water containing a lot of aluminum. This development gives even more credibility to the theory that aluminum is related to Alzheimer's disease. According to one story in *Lancet* (2:116), a 44-year-old man who received kidney dialysis in an area where the tap water had a high content of aluminum developed almost complete memory loss during the time of treatment. However, he became able to remember normally again after 259 mg of aluminum was removed from his body. (See the next article, "Aluminum in Our Water," for more information.)

Of additional interest, scientists have found that animals fed aluminum for several months eventually die with brain damage similar to that found in humans with Alzheimer's disease. Also, medical researchers have discovered that brain tissue from people dying with Alzheimer's contains much higher levels of aluminum than the brain tissue of mentally normal people of the same age who die from other causes.

In view of all this, a physician writing to the editor of the *New England Journal of Medicine* (303:164) suggests that gradual build-up of aluminum in the brain may well account for the gross loss of memory and judgment characteristic of Alzheimer's.

The reason why the onset of the disease is delayed in most cases until the age of about 80, however, has never been plausibly explained. At last, though, in light of research reported in the *Lancet* (2:1227), we may be closer to the answer.

Aluminum, it was found, not only damages the brain directly, but also harms it by lowering the effectiveness of the blood brain barrier (BBB), a layer of tissue that normally acts as a protective coating between the bloodstream and the brain's nerve tissues. Normally, the BBB keeps toxic body waste products from getting out of the blood into the nervous system. When the kidneys age and become less efficient at ridding the body of waste products, particularly those derived from protein breakdown, the concentration of these substances in the bloodstream increases, and, if the BBB is no longer intact, they are able to get into the brain and poison it.

Significantly, it was discovered that one of these toxic waste products causes memory loss and selectively damages parts of the brain that are most affected by Alzheimer's disease. Thus, aided and abetted by the aging of the kidneys, aluminum helps to bring on Alzheimer's in two ways: by directly poisoning the brain, and by injuring the BBB so that other poisons can damage the brain as well.

Aluminum in Our Water

To survive after both kidneys have failed, one must either have a kidney graft or be treated by dialysis regularly for the rest of one's life. Dialysis nowadays usually involves rinsing out the peritoneal cavity (the space between the intestines and the abdominal wall) with several gallons of fluid two or three times a week to remove body wastes which would normally be carried away in the urine.

Several thousand people have been dialyzed for many years, most of them without serious complications. Infection, of course, is always a threat, but can be treated with antibiotics. A much more serious complication, though, is permanent brain damage with mental deterioration, known as dialysis dementia. This, according to *Lancet* (2:190), occurs only in people who have undergone dialysis in certain geographical areas in Europe and America.

A mystery until recently, dialysis dementia (almost exactly like Alzheimer's disease, but occurring at any age) is now known to be caused by traces of aluminum in the water from which the dialysis fluid is prepared. Aluminum is absorbed into the patient's body at the time of dialysis and poisons the brain.

Kidney failure patients undergoing dialysis in localities where there is a lot of aluminum in the tap water ultimately suffer memory loss and other signs of brain damage. Even young people undergoing dialysis have this problem, but the effects may be reversible if treated early enough. The effect of long-standing aluminum build-up in older people, however, could well become permanent.

Even though aluminum is used for water purification in many cities, including all those where dialysis dementia has occurred, most of us do not get dementia from it (at least not early in life) because we drink only a pint or two of water a day. In contrast, when the water contains a lot of aluminum, kidney failure patients cannot avoid absorbing a very much larger amount of it from the several gallons of fluid which must be used in dialysis two or three times every week.

Many municipal water companies employ an aluminum-containing chemical get for water purification. Even though these companies may argue that mere "traces" of aluminum get into our drinking water, these amounts are nevertheless sufficient to bring on hip fractures and dementia in young people (in their teens, 20s and 30s) who must use large volumes of water for dialysis. Just think what this water could do to the rest of us more slowly over a lifetime!

Concerned and politically active readers might wish to ask about this in their hometowns and invite their water companies to discuss alternatives. Some major city water companies have already started purifying their water successfully without aluminum.

Aluminum also gets into our water is through acid rain. Sulfur released into the atmosphere from industrial smokestacks ultimately falls back onto the earth's surface again hundreds or thousands of miles away in the form of sulfuric acid, which not only kills fish and vegetable life but also threatens man, the *Lancet* (1:616) reports. The acid reacts with substances in the soil, breaking them down from harmless complex molecules into simpler substances, some of which are salts of toxic metals, such as aluminum, mercury, and lead, which get into the surface water that we drink.

Although it is understood that these metals kill fish, there is still a lot of reluctance to accept the idea that they could be harmful to human beings as well. But since there is always the possibility of this danger for us when we drink surface water, we could try to help ourselves by drinking ground water from deep wells instead.

Aluminum Awareness

As pointed out in the previous articles, the idea that parts of our brain are gradually being destroyed by traces of aluminum that we absorb from our food and drinking water can no longer be easily dismissed. Aluminum is not only used by many of our cities for water purification but also is an ingredient in a wide variety of medicines, cosmetics, and foods. In fact, it is rather frightening to discover just how widely aluminum is used.

It is disturbing to find aluminum in so many cake mixes, salad dressings, pickles, baking powder (not baking soda), and processed cheese. Some (but not all) ready-to-sprinkle grated Parmesan cheese products (and other grated cheeses) contain an aluminum salt to enhance pourability. There is also an aluminum compound in several of the most widely used brands of table salt (to help it retain pourability under moist conditions). Fortunately, some brands of "sea salt" remain aluminum-free. These are available in most large supermarkets.

Many lipsticks, skin creams, and lotions contain aluminum. Because it is inexpensive, light and fluffy, and imparts a creamy smooth texture to their products, manufacturers regard aluminum as a good "filler." Alum, please note, is also an aluminum compound.

As the main active ingredient, an aluminum compound is also included in most antiperspirants (sprays, sticks, and roll-ons). The compound temporarily poisons sweat glands, thereby providing fairly long-lasting dryness. For the same reason, presumably, aluminum features in many feminine hygiene products.

A large number of common medicines, including several brands of aspirin, contain aluminum. One should try to avoid any medications containing salts of aluminum. Since there are usually aluminum-free equivalents for them, we suggest you read medicine bottle labels and, if necessary, discuss this with your pharmacist. Fortunately, the marketplace offers alternative products that are aluminum-free and, by reading labels, we can protect ourselves.

Other ways we can avoid unnecessary aluminum intake is by discarding our aluminum pots, pans and percolators and by drinking from bottles rather than from cans.

Aluminum and Iron

Hematologists (physicians specialized in disorders of the blood) at Heidelberg in Germany have encountered several dialysis patients with typical iron-deficiency anemia who nevertheless had a perfectly adequate intake of iron. Reporting their findings in the *Lancet* (1:1390), these physicians managed to track down the cause of this seemingly incongruous manifestation of iron deficiency "amid plenty." Aluminum was the culprit.

Aluminum, apparently, accumulates in the bone marrow cells responsible for red blood cell formation and so occupies them that it is no longer possible for them to absorb and utilize iron. Thus, although absorbed into the body quite normally, the iron cannot be used any more for red blood cell production. Here is one more example of the sinister biological effects of aluminum.

Aluminum can slowly accumulate in the tissues over a lifetime to bring about both thinning of the bones with fractures and brain damage. Furthermore, as we have noted in the previous articles, an increasing number of experts on aging believe that aluminum build-up in the brain is at least a contributory cause, if not the main one, of Alzheimer's disease.

Zinc and Alzheimer's

Whereas brain poisoning by the gradual accumulation of aluminum in the brain may well be one of the causes of Alzheimer's disease, a new theory is that zinc shortage may be important, too. According to the *Lancet* (1:8213), zinc is a vital component of enzymes (chemical machinery) that repair worn out cells in the brain. It is suggested that Alzheimer's dementia begins when these enzymes, for one reason or another, no longer get all the zinc they need.

It is important to note, however, that our dietary intake of metals needs to be well balanced. According to the *Journal of the American Medical Association* (245:1528), too much zinc interferes with copper absorption, another essential metal. Copper deficiency, in turn, results in anemia and raises the blood cholesterol sufficiently to bring on atherosclerosis.

Excess zinc, some arthritis experts think, directly injures the lining of blood vessels and may also, in some people, convert mild cases of the chronic disease lupus erythematosus into more serious ones. They cannot prove this but have seen several patients in whom the associated events strongly suggests that it is so.

How much zinc is too much? No one really knows. Nevertheless, Harrison's *Textbook of Medicine* (9th.ed.p.381) tells us that zinc in daily doses of 100 mg or more interferes with certain enzymes and counteracts some treatments for hypertension. Accordingly, until we know more about it, those who take extra zinc would be wise to keep the dosage well below 100 mg and not take it every day.

Alzheimer's Disease Can Be Misdiagnosed!

Loss of memory for recent events, mental slowness, depression, dementia, deafness, weight loss, weakness, "rheumatism," constipation, and incontinence in an elderly person are usually regarded as unavoidable features of aging. Some older people who have these symptoms, however, may be suffering from hypothyroidism (abnormally low hormone output by the thyroid gland), the *Western Journal of Medicine* (143:643) reports.

In young people, mental slowness nearly always arouses suspicion of thyroid disease, but in older people it is usually blamed on Alzheimer's disease. Hypothyroidism, of course, is a much more desirable diagnosis since, unlike senile dementia (Alzheimer's disease), it can be treated, and, with thyroid hormone given by mouth, most patients rapidly recover.

Recognizing this disease, however, may be difficult since its features are often not typical in old age. Nevertheless, hypothyroidism is one of the more common ailments of the elderly and is known as "the great masquerader of geriatrics." It may even be the cause of dementia in a large percentage of cases. Since hypothyroidism is often due to an iodine deficiency, we can help to prevent it by using iodized salt and by taking a daily tablet of kelp, a seaweed product that contains natural iodine.

ANEMIA

Anemia — the Tip of an Iceberg?

Anemia is the term applied to any condition in which the concentration of hemoglobin (the red oxygen-carrying pigment) in the blood is below normal. It is rarely a disease in itself and is nearly always caused by something else, such as bleeding, a deficiency, kidney trouble, an infection, or cancer. So important is this point that *Hospital Practice* recently saw fit to highlight it in an editorial.

Most anemias, fortunately, turn out to be nothing more serious than iron deficiency, a condition that can usually be corrected with medication. Some cases of iron deficiency, however, result from bleeding — the cause of which is not always easy to find. A bleeding gastric ulcer is usually obvious because of associated indigestion and abdominal pain, but bleeding from cancer of the colon can be without symptoms until the tumor is far advanced. In civilized countries, most iron-deficiency anemia is caused by heavy menstrual bleeding in women who don't take enough iron to make up for it. In the tropics, iron deficiency more often results from intestinal worms, which steal the patient's blood.

Other types of anemia are due to decreased production of red cells (which carry the hemoglobin in the blood) or to an increase in their rate of destruction. Every day, about 1 percent of our red blood cells wear out and are replaced by new ones from the bone marrow, and anemia results whenever this balance is disturbed. Any one of a great number of conditions, including infections (such as syphilis, tuberculosis, or malaria), thyroid trouble, kidney problems, leukemia, poisons, or dietary deficiencies can increase the destruction or decrease the production of red cells.

Anemia, therefore, is like the tip of an iceberg and must always be taken seriously as a clue to illness. Simple iron and vitamin remedies should not be used in its treatment routinely but only after the major serious causes have been ruled out. If you become anemic, your physician may need to run many tests on you. Cooperate fully, because it's in your best interests.

Iron Deficiency and Unusual Dietary Cravings

Iron deficiency can cause a condition called pica, which is the compulsive eating of almost anything, including dirt or clay (geophagia), starch (amylophagia), and ice (pagophagia). Not just an occasional zany impulse, pica is the continuous obsessive craving for the unconventional dietary experience.

A case reported in the *Annals of Internal Medicine* (94:660) illustrates a potential complication. A 74-year-old woman with iron deficiency had a craving for magnesium carbonate, which she ate several times a day. In quantity, magnesium acts as a laxative and causes the too rapid transit of food through the intestines, with failure of absorption of dietary ingredients, including iron. So, in this case, as in many others, iron deficiency caused pica and thereby made itself worse.

Pica and its complications usually respond rapidly to an injection of iron.

Tea Drinking as a Cause of Anemia?

Many things can influence the amount of iron we absorb and retain from our food. If we lose blood or become anemic for any reason, iron absorption usually increases, so that when iron is in short supply, we compensate by absorbing it more efficiently. Our ability to absorb increased amounts of iron when necessary, however, is variable, a human inconsistency which has always puzzled hematologists.

Now, according to the *New England Journal of Medicine*, tea-drinking may help to explain some of these differences in iron absorption. It has been found, for instance, that tea reduces iron absorption from food by as much as 95 percent. Whereas in some diseases this could be helpful because there is already too much iron in the body, if you have a problem absorbing iron, or there is inadequate iron in your diet (most vegetarians need to take iron), you may want to limit the amount of tea you drink.

Iron Deficiency Correction

Anemic nomads in Africa suddenly came down with tuberculosis and other infections when iron was added to their food. Iron deficiency, it seems, had been protecting them by preventing bacterial growth in their tissues.

Now, according to *Pediatrics*, the same sort of thing has been observed in the United States. Adding extra iron to infant formula, it has been found, encourages growth of contaminant bacteria in the milk. Fortunately, the iron in human milk, unlike that in cow's milk, is bound to a special protein and is not available to bacteria. If mothers nurse their babies and take sufficient iron in their food, their babies will get all the iron they need in the safest possible way.

ANOREXIA NERVOSA

The Seriousness of Anorexia Nervosa

Anorexia nervosa is a dangerous illness brought on by abnormally depleted diets, and its victims are usually young women who have an obsessive desire to be thin. Typically, a young woman loses so much weight that she becomes skeletal in appearance, and eventually, so weak that she has to remain in bed. The weakness can be so profound that eating enough to remain alive becomes progressively more difficult so that the patient may ultimately die.

With the current emphasis on slimness, anorexia nervosa has become much more common and may now affect about 0.4 percent (one in 250) of adolescent females in Western countries, the *Annals of Internal Medicine* (102:49) reports.

Even though its origin may be largely "psychological," it must not be taken lightly because, according to the *Annals*, the death rate can be as high as 30 percent. The cause of death, a sudden heart rhythm disturbance, is similar, if not identical, to that seen in people taking a liquid protein diet.

Zinc and Anorexia Nervosa

Probably the most difficult aspect of the disease anorexia nervosa is that patients start out by dieting rather strenuously and then, after losing a lot of weight, find that they cannot get back to normal again even if they try. Getting these people to absorb food, even after tube feeding, is not always successful.

Now, according to the *Lancet* (2:350), one patient, at least, has responded dramatically to supplemental zinc, and on the basis of this case, there is hope that zinc will prove beneficial to others.

Zinc deficiency, it is well known, greatly impairs our sense of taste and smell, thereby markedly reducing the appetite. Furthermore, zinc deficiency probably also impairs the absorptive functions of the intestine, the *Lancet* (2:350) reports, hence explaining the lack of success of tube feedings. It is understandable that as patients become zinc deficient as the result of their dieting, the deficiency makes the situation worse by depriving them of any further desire for food.

For more information about zinc (the dangers of both the deficiency and the overdosage), see the articles about this mineral in the section *Vitamin, Mineral Dosages*.

ARTHRITIS

Gouty Arthritis and Vitamin A

Although gout is known to result from uric acid crystallizing out of the blood into the joints, no one knows why only certain joints are involved, or why the disease varies in intensity from time to time regardless of how carefully one avoids foods that raise the uric acid blood level. Experts have suggested, therefore, that other unknown factors may trigger attacks of gout as well.

A rheumatologist from one of the major university medical centers recently wrote to the editor of *Lancet* (1:1181) suggesting that vitamin A and alcohol may be additional factors that, working together with uric acid, could bring on gouty arthritis in certain joints. Just a slight excess of vitamin A in the diet makes the blood uric acid rise much higher than it otherwise would, the rheumatologist reports. Furthermore, he states, quite normal doses of vitamin A can act like overdoses if, in addition, one takes several alcoholic drinks regularly every day.

Even by itself, when regularly taken in excess, vitamin A can cause pain in the feet, ankles, wrists, or shoulders. This is due to swelling and thickening of the bones, especially at their surfaces, along with calcium deposition in the ligaments and muscles attached to them. Since these changes can mimic gout, the rheumatologist suggests, many people who have been told that they have gouty arthritis may really be suffering from the effects of moderate but regularly taken doses of vitamin A and alcohol.

Rather than just taking gout medication, therefore, such persons might do better if they also reduced their vitamin A intake to avoid overdosage and took fewer alcoholic drinks as well.

Gout Aggravated by Chicken Gravy

According to the U.S. Dept. of Agriculture, there is more hypoxanthine (a chemical that stirs up gout) in chicken meat than in almost any other food. Roasted or broiled chicken is fairly safe because, according to *Modern Medicine* (50#3:24), most of the hypoxanthine leaves the meat with the juices during cooking.

Nevertheless, fried chicken or roasted chicken that has been basted with its own gravy, like chicken soup, is best avoided by those who suffer from gout.

Iron and Arthritis

Rheumatoid arthritis, rare in the Third World but common in the U.S.A., may in some cases be at least partly due to an excess of iron. According to a theory proposed in *Lancet* (2:1142), iron deficiency, brought on in poor countries by malnutrition and intestinal parasites, may help to prevent arthritis by damping down inflammation. The inflammatory response, besides being part of our natural defenses against infection and trauma, can be very damaging if it lasts too long, and some types of arthritis seem to be due to inflammation entirely.

Adding credibility to this theory is the observation that rheumatoid arthritis is relatively uncommon in young women. After the menopause, however, when women stop losing blood (and iron) with menses, they become much more prone (like men) to it. Patients with rheumatoid arthritis, further-more, have higher iron blood levels when their joints are swollen and painful than when their arthritis is "in remission."

According to *Harrison's Principles of Internal Medicine* (9th ed:488) excessive iron intake for many years, besides making the skin look bronzed, may injure the heart (bringing on failure), and cause damage to the liver, pancreas (bringing on diabetes), and, of course, the joints. Furthermore, there is a growing conviction among physicians that, except during childhood and pregnancy and in premenopausal women, there is no need for iron in more than maintenance amounts, unless it must be given, temporarily, for the treatment of anemia. One must be careful, therefore, not to continue taking iron in therapeutic doses for any longer than it is needed.

Salmon Oil for Arthritis?

Two arthritis specialists, working independently of one another at different medical schools (Albany Medical College, N.Y., and Harvard University), have both had good results with salmon oil capsules (Maxepa) when studying their effect in patients with rheumatoid arthritis.

While receiving Maxepa (15-20 capsules daily), the patients experienced both fewer painful joints and less morning stiffness, changes that did not occur when the patients (without knowing it) received capsules of a placebo instead. These findings were statistically significant, *Medical World News* (27#13:9) reports. While none of their patients became completely symptom-free during these clinical trials, the doctors pointed out that the treatment periods were very brief (just a few weeks), and that much longer trials will be needed to determine just how active Maxepa really is against arthritis.

Maxepa is technically a "food" rather than a drug, and it has been taken by a very large number of people for many years for the reduction of cholesterol blood levels and the prevention of hardening of the arteries. It is an over-the-counter product marketed by R.P.Scherer Corporation, P. O. Box 5600, Clearwater, Fla. 33518, and it has never been reported to cause side effects of any kind. However, Maxepa has not yet been approved by the Food and Drug Administration for treatment of arthritis.

Arthritis from Food Allergy

After 11 years of pain, swelling, and stiffness of her joints, symptoms believed by all concerned to be typical of rheumatoid arthritis, a 52-year-old woman was found to be really suffering from an allergy to milk, *Arthritis and Rheumatism* (29:220) reports. Everyone was surprised when milk (and everything made from it) was removed from her diet, and her arthritic symptoms went away. So long as she went without milk, the swelling, pain and, stiffness of her joints (worst in her hands) totally disappeared.

Proof of a cause-and-effect relationship between her arthritis and milk allergy was obtained when, from time to time, she was given capsules of what she thought was medication but which, in fact, contained powdered milk. On each of these occasions, without exception, she experienced a temporary return of the arthritis. The report concludes with the thought that an unrecognized allergy of some sort might be the cause of arthritis in many other people. It would certainly be worth looking for when, as is so often the case, rheumatoid arthritis fails to respond well to the usual treatments.

Anti-Arthritis Drugs Affect the Brain

According to a report in *Arthritis and Rheumatism* (25:1013), memory loss, inability to concentrate, and changes in personality are being encountered in elderly people who take one of the nonsteroidal anti-inflammatory drugs (NSAIDs) for arthritis. All of these drugs relieve pain, whether or not it is due to arthritis, and must therefore have some effect on nerve tissue.

Accordingly, it is not too surprising that they can affect the brain as well. Some of the most widely used drugs of this type include Clinoral, Motrin, Nalfon, Naprosyn, Rufen, and Tolectin. These effects have appeared after about two months of treatment and have disappeared completely within two weeks after the causative drug has been discontinued.

Because mental changes are so often ascribed to "senility," be on the lookout for this side effect. Aspirin, as well, can do this, *Clinical Pharmacology and Therapeutics* (32:362) reports, but only with very high doses that are far greater than most people use.

Ice Packs for Arthritic Knees

Despite medication, people with arthritis are frequently disabled with pain, especially in the knees. Heat is then usually applied, but, more often than not, it provides little relief. Nevertheless, heat is often continued with the hope that it will at least reduce stiffness. When all else fails, ice bags are then sometimes tried.

Frustrated by their failures, Oregon University arthritis specialists recently broke with tradition by using ice first, instead of heat. By getting their patients to hold six ice cubes in a plastic bag both above and below the knee for 20 minutes three times a day, they reduced pain and, as the weeks passed, improved their patients' mobility and increased the duration of their sleep. Although cold therapy takes getting used to, reports the *Journal of the American Medical Association* (246:317), patients who start it, without exception, do not want to stop.

ASTHMA

Asthma: Know the Danger Signals

An article entitled "Fatal Asthma" in the *New England Journal of Medicine* (314:423) reminds us of the need, at all times, to be alert to oncoming attacks of this disease.

One way of getting an early warning that all is not well is to encourage asthma patients to take daily readings of their own respiratory flow rate (the speed at which air flows in and out of the mouth during breathing with the nostrils closed), using the simple whistle-like instrument known as a spirometer. Most allergy specialists will be pleased to show their patients how to do this.

This test can also warn of the need for extra medication and medical help, which is often put off until there is dangerous distress. When, in spite of these measures, patients suddenly find themselves in respiratory difficulty, it is essential that they do everything possible to prevent their airways from becoming dried out, since dried mucus in the passageways of the chest not only chokes them up but also irritates them as well. This irritation and choking, in turn, triggers bouts of coughing and causes them to go into typical asthmatic spasm.

A way of helping to prevent this is to drink a lot of water when an asthma attack seems to be on the way. The victim should sit down and keep sipping from a large glassful of warm (not hot) water until the entire glassful has been swallowed in about 15 minutes. As soon as this has been done, another glassful of warm water should be taken during the next 15 minutes. In this way, the victim drinks about one pint of water in half an hour, a procedure that can abort many attacks.

Asthma victims should also learn to discipline themselves during attacks and breathe more deeply and slowly. Usually, because of their anxiety, they breathe too rapidly and ineffectively, thereby merely drying out the upper airways, exhausting themselves, and making matters much worse than they need be. Many deaths could be avoided if asthma patients knew when they were getting into trouble and then got themselves admitted to a hospital without delay.

Asthma without Wheezing

Usually, asthma attacks begin with coughing and wheezing and then progress to severe difficulty in breathing. Wheezing and shortness of breath are such notable features of these attacks that, without them, coughing alone is rarely suspected of being asthmatic in nature. Nevertheless, there is now proof that just plain coughing, particularly if it lasts longer than a week, can be due to a mild form of asthma. According to the *New England Journal of Medicine*, this can be put to the test by giving the patient asthma medicine. If the patient stops coughing, the diagnosis of asthma is confirmed.

This may not seem very exciting, but it can save a lot of money and time. Until now, people with chronic cough have usually undergone lengthy and expensive tests for lung cancer, tuberculosis, etc. Only when those more serious illnesses had been ruled out was it safe for physicians to consider less serious causes such as asthma. Now, knowing that they can detect asthmatic coughing quickly and reliably merely by giving medicine, they can do this first.

Chronic cough is most likely due to asthma when there is

a family history of allergy. Nevertheless, anyone with a cough lasting several weeks should seek medical attention.

Vitamin C for Asthma

Perhaps suggested by the observation that 19th century sailors who had scurvy stopped wheezing when they ate citrus fruits, researchers have found that 500 mg of vitamin C relaxes the air passages of patients with exercise-induced asthma.

According to their report in the *Journal of the American Medical Association* (245:548), this small protective effect (about 15 percent) may nevertheless be enough to stimulate the development of a new class of drugs for this condition. Further research is proceeding on patients who develop asthma on exposure to cotton and wool fibers.

Aspirin-Induced Asthma

Attacks of aspirin-induced asthma are so long-lasting, so resistant to treatment, and have such a high fatality rate that anyone who has ever had asthma (whether or not they are known to be sensitive to aspirin) should avoid the drug permanently.

Since asthma and other allergies tend to run in families, *Modern Medicine* (49#8:103) warns, it is also advisable for anyone with an aspirin-sensitive relative to avoid aspirin. This also applies to indomethacin, another pain-relieving medication, because there is often cross-hypersensitivity between these drugs. Acetaminophen, another efficient pain reliever, can be used instead.

Because aspirin is so often just one of several ingredients in a medication, read the complete formula and be on the lookout not only for the word "aspirin" but also for its alternative names, acetylsalicylic acid and A.S.A.

Asthma and Storms

So many people have had attacks of asthma at the same time in some cities that the term "asthma epidemic" has been justifiably used. Smog from automobile exhaust or industrial pollution has been the obvious cause in many of these epidemics, but for some of them (New Orleans and New York, for example), no obvious triggering cause could be identified.

Now, however, it seems that fungus spore fragments and particles of pollen too small to be easily detected by usual methods, may be the culprits for these mysterious asthma epidemics, the *Lancet* (1:1079) reports. Tiny allergy-provoking particles are produced during storms when rain beats on puffballs, other types of fungi, and upon seeding grass.

The damp air after storms may be a veritable allergenic soup, especially if the humidity remains high and has not necessarily been "washed" and purified by the rain, even if the larger dust particles have been settled, and the air smells fresh and clean. If there is no wind to blow the dampness away, it would therefore be wise for asthmatics to stay indoors for a day after heavy rain during the summer and fall.

Coffee and Asthma

The belief expressed by many asthmatics that coffee drinking can help relieve their attacks has been given scientific support by a study that has just been reported in the *Medical World News* (24#23:21). Theobromine, a natural chemical of the coffee plant, affects the body in almost the same way as theophylline, one of the most commonly used drugs for asthma.

Not surprisingly, therefore, asthmatics who have taken a normal dose of theophylline experience unusually intense side effects from that medication if they drink coffee at the same time. This, of course, is due to the additive side effects on the body of the two very similar chemical compounds. Asthmatics who drank three cups of coffee as well as taking their medicine experienced nervousness, headache, palpitations, and upset stomach.

These were the side effects that they might get with theophylline anyway, but they were much more intense than the asthmatic patients expected them to be. Tea and cola drinks, even though containing similar chemical stimulants, are not strong enough in this respect to produce additive effects.

BACK PAIN

Back Trouble in Older Women

In older women, a loss of calcium from the skeleton (osteoporosis) causes broken bones. Fractured hips are a well-known result of this but it is not so widely recognized that many other types of fracture are associated with it, too. Actually, compression fractures of the vertebrae (spinal bones), with loss of body height and rounding of the back, are probably the most common.

In X-rays taken from the side, an affected vertebra (which

is normally cylindrical) appears wedge-shaped. This is because only the front part of the vertebra collapses under the weight of the upper trunk; the back part holds up because it is supported by the attached bony arch that surrounds the spinal cord.

People with compression fracture of the spine, according to the *Mayo Clinic Proceedings* (57:699), most commonly complain of backache, with pain radiating down and around the side to the front. Depending upon how quickly the bone collapses, this pain may come on gradually or suddenly. Sometimes it is more noticeable in front than behind and may then be wrongly attributed to heart or gall bladder troubles.

Many women adjust to chronic backache but temporarily experience additional disabling pain every time another vertebra collapses. With each fracture, the *Proceedings* recommends, the woman should stay in bed for about three weeks (getting up only to the toilet) to take the weight off the bone while it starts to heal. Even when there is already loss of height and spinal curvature, a specially fitted back brace can be most helpful in relieving pain and in preventing further deformity. Forward bending to lift things must be avoided since it puts further strain on the front of weakened vertebrae.

Calcium carbonate (one gram), vitamin D (400 units), and a long walk every day help to preserve the strength of the bones. Additionally, many physicians now also give women who have just gone through the menopause small daily doses of estrogen.

Spinal Manipulation

Because spinal manipulation involves so much physical contact between patient and doctor, critics of this treatment attribute its success to the placebo effect of psychological support. Others question its safety. Carefully looking into the pros and cons of spinal manipulation, a team of physical medicine experts has studied this procedure in 1,880 patients at the Back Clinic of the Irvine Medical Center, California.

Publishing their findings in the *Journal of the American Medical Association* (245:1835), they demonstrated rather convincingly that pain relief produced by spinal manipulation is greater and more immediate than that resulting from either massage or medication. Furthermore, although there have been occasional reports of injury, they concluded that lower back manipulation is quite safe when performed by qualified practitioners. Please note that this applies only to lower spinal manipulation. Neck manipulation, an entirely different procedure, is inherently more dangerous.

The Irvine investigators also observed that certain types of patients should not receive spinal manipulation. These include pregnant women and anyone with osteoporosis (thinning of the bones, e.g., after the menopause), osteomyelitis (bone infection), metabolic disorders of bone (e.g., rickets or bony changes secondary to kidney, thyroid or pituitary disorders, etc.), fractures, cancer, ankylosing spondylitis (progressive arthritis with fusing together of the spinal bones), intervertebral disc displacement, or narrowing of the arteries feeding the spine.

Prolapsed Intervertebral Disk

Ultimately, after many backache attacks, with pain down the back of the leg, people who have a prolapsed intervertebral disk (also known as a herniated disk) may need to have the disk removed. It causes pain by pressing on nerve roots in the spine.

The removal can be done by an injection into the disk to dissolve it away, or by an operation. Less severe attacks usually respond to a week or two of rest and medication, followed by special exercises.

However, *Modern Medicine* (52#11:119) reports, the most important thing is to find the position of maximum relief. For the majority of people, this involves lying on the floor with both knees pointing at the ceiling and with the lower legs resting horizontally on the seat of a chair. Others will need to experiment and find their own position of maximum comfort. Because this takes the pressure of the disk off the nerves, it is the first step needed for obtaining relief.

Initially, it may be necessary to maintain this position almost continuously for some days, but, later, when the victim gets better and goes back to work, it will be helpful if this position is adopted for at least 30 minutes during the day (it is better to do this for five minutes six times daily than to do it only once for 30 minutes). It is also important to avoid any positions and movements that bring on the pain. Medications help to lessen the pain but are less important than bodily position and rest (waterbeds should not be used).

After the pain subsides, the patient should start exercises to develop the muscles of the back and lower abdomen. This helps to prevent the lax and excessive movements that allow a disk to prolapse. Exercises that cause pain, however, must be stopped immediately and only those that can be performed in comfort should be continued. Lastly, one must learn to sit and lift correctly to avoid reinjuring the back.

The Danger of Weight Lifting

The sport of weight lifting can be dangerous, especially for young people before their bones have fully developed at about the age of 21, and causes damage particularly to their knees, spine, and shoulders. Even in the fully mature, spinal disk problems may be bought on by heavy lifting. Transient elevations of blood pressure, with burst blood vessels, and even blackouts (resulting in dropped weights, which can cause injury, too) are additional potential dangers.

Weight training, is not to be confused with weight lifting. It is not a sport but, according to the *Physician and Sportsmedicine* (11#3:157), a method of training that involves full-range, repetitive muscular movements against submaximal resistance, usually by moving weights suspended by ropes over pulleys. The "load" or resistance is individualized and gradually increased as muscular strength improves, but at no time exceeds that person's maximum capability, a safeguard that prevents strain. Weight training is therefore much safer than weight lifting for people of all ages.

BLINDNESS

Transient Blindness, a Warning of Stroke

Episodes of blindness, lasting up to five minutes and involving part or all of the visual field, are often a sign of decreased blood flow to the eye or to its nerve connections inside the brain. This is a warning of impending stroke.

About one in five persons so affected, according to the *Lancet* (1:838), will show X-ray evidence of a narrowed artery in the neck. Due to atherosclerosis (cholesterol deposits), the narrowed part of the artery can usually be removed, thereby improving the blood flow and helping to prevent a stroke.

Whether or not surgery can be performed, all other possible means of preventing stroke should be employed in such cases. These measures should include keeping the blood pressure down to normal and taking a medication such as aspirin in doses that slow the blood clotting mechanism.

First Aid for Sudden Blindness

Vision is lost instantly when blood stops flowing through the arteries which feed the retina (the light-sensing surface in the back of the eye). Depending on the size of artery and the amount of retina deprived of blood supply, visual loss varies all the way from a small blind spot to total blindness in the affected eye.

The usual cause of this sudden but painless blindness is a small blood clot wedging in a branch of the retinal artery that is already narrowed by atherosclerosis. This dams the artery and stops its blood flow. People sometimes experience this type of blindness only for a few minutes until the clot breaks up or drifts away from the narrowed part of the artery. Vision, of course, returns only if blood flow is restored soon enough — about one and three-fourths hours is usually the limit.

Now, according to the *Journal of the American Medical Association*, people can help themselves when this sudden blindness strikes by gently massaging the affected eye with on-and-off pressure applied over the closed upper eyelid about once every 15 seconds. The pressure should be firm but not enough to hurt.

Even though results cannot be guaranteed, this procedure, which is analogous to cardiopulmonary resuscitation, may disperse the clot and is surely worth trying. Recent eye surgery, of course, would contraindicate it. Also, when the afflicted person has diabetes, or a feeling of tightness, pain or any other hint of bleeding inside the eye, this first aid treatment must not be used.

Early Warning of Retinal Detachment

By knowing about the first signs of retinal detachment, we greatly improve our chances of getting early enough treatment to prevent blindness. The most important signs include the sudden appearance of "floaters" (small shadowy shapes like flies or spider webs constantly dangling in our field of vision no matter where we look) and spontaneous flickers or flashes of light (like fireflies or sheet lightning) which are most noticeable in the evening and in the morning before daylight. As more and more retina becomes detached, a growing curtain of darkness seems to surround the things one looks at and which one can still see clearly.

Tragically, because the center of the retina is usually the last part to become detached, the ability to read and watch TV, etc., is preserved intact until the last moment before total blindness occurs. This misleads people into believing that their symptoms are not serious. According to *Geriatrics* (365#4:87), retinal detachment is most likely to occur in people with myopia (nearsightedness), high blood pressure, or diabetes.

Blindness Prevention for Diabetics

Because loss of vision is so common in diabetes, all victims of this disease should have their eyes examined at least once a year by an ophthalmologist (an M.D. who has specialized in diseases of the eyes). Tragically, however, about 50 percent of diabetics lose their vision needlessly because they do not follow this advice, the *British Medical Journal* (293.1508) reports.

About 10 million Americans are diabetic and 400,000 of them have macular edema, an abnormality of the retina (light-sensitive layer in the back of the eye) that slowly produces blindness if not halted by laser treatment. The macula is that part of the retina concerned with seeing details, as in reading and recognizing faces. When macular vision is lost, one becomes "legally blind" and can appreciate only the movement of big objects and the difference between light and dark.

A diabetic loses his macular vision when blood leaks from his retinal blood vessels and accumulates in the macula, compressing and destroying its visual nerve endings. Detected in time, however, macular edema can usually be prevented from worsening, or at least slowed. Laser beam treatment coagulates leaking blood vessels in the macula and thus seals them. This is expensive (about $1,500-$2,000 per eye), but is covered by Medicare and private insurers.

Since early cases of macular edema are often symptomless, and advanced cases may be impossible to treat, a regular program of examinations by an ophthalmologist should be begun before any visual loss occurs. The penalty for not doing this can be blindness.

Too many diabetics rely upon the family doctor, internist, or optometrist to advise them when to seek an ophthalmologist's help. By that time, unfortunately, it is usually too late.

Stated simply, the ophthalmologist looks for the earliest possible signs of leaking blood vessels in the retina. To do this, he employs drops to dilate the pupils and, after injecting fluorescent dye, takes retinal pictures. Leaking vessels show up as patches of retinal fluorescence and can be sealed off with a laser beam. The whole procedure may be carried out in the doctor's office. If diabetics wish to preserve their vision, nothing less than this type of retinal blood vessel monitoring will do.

Preventable Blindness

In senile macular degeneration (SMD), new blood vessels grow over the retina (the light-sensing layer in the back of the eye), distorting it so that it no longer functions properly. Although SMD accounts for nearly all new cases of blindness in people over 65, its cause remains unknown.

Nevertheless, physicians working at the National Eye Institute have made an exciting announcement. A brief session in the doctor's office with about 10 minutes of laser beam treatment usually stops the blood vessel proliferation and restores normal vision in over 80 percent of cases. Most of the remainder benefit, too, but partially. Many people need this treatment repeatedly.

The researchers announcing this advance in *Archives of Ophthalmology* (100:911) make it clear that, to benefit SMD patients must obtain laser treatment soon after the onset of symptoms. If they wait too long, irreversible damage will already have been done. To catch SMD recurrences early enough, the researchers urge, all victims should test their own vision daily with an Amsler grid (which they can get from an ophthalmologist), and report changes right away.

Lenses Correct Color Blindness

Color blindness can now usually be improved with a red-tinted contact lens. Although this treatment does not work for the few people who totally lack red-green discrimination, it works well enough for the majority, who have partial impairment, that they are able to pass Federal Aviation Administration tests.

Known as the X-Chrom lens, it is worn in only one eye, preferably the non-dominant one, with a regular untinted lens on the other side. Before its effect becomes optimal, according to the *Journal of the American Medical Association* (244:2457), a tinted lens may need to be worn for several weeks.

BLOOD PRESSURE— AGGRAVATORS

Salt and Blood Pressure

To help millions of Americans who must limit their salt (sodium chloride) intake, more and more food processors are declaring the salt content of their products in their labeling. Consumers should be aware that the two-letter symbol "Na" is an abbreviation of the Latin word "natrium," sodium's international chemical name.

They should also realize that monosodium glutamate (MSG), sodium citrate or nitrate, etc., are no less dangerous, so far as sodium content is concerned, than common salt. Baking soda is extremely rich in sodium; baking powder is less so, although still high. A Food and Drug Administration *Drug Bulletin* (13#3:25) reveals that diet soft drinks contain more sodium than do the regular ones, and that club soda contains the most. Of alcoholic drinks, beer contains the most salt. Among cheeses, the Swiss types contain the least. Beware of prepared desserts and puddings and especially of chocolate pudding. Many non-prescription drugs, most notably the antacids, contain a lot of sodium.

Sometimes foods which we think are healthy actually contain more salt than we realize. Although advertisements for Cheerios state that this cereal is recommended by pediatricians as the ideal solid food for toddlers, a letter to the editor of the *Lancet* (1:1052) points out that its high salt content makes it unsafe for young people. Containing nearly a third of a gram of salt per one-ounce serving, Cheerios is actually saltier than most "salty" foods, such as potato chips. Wheaties, another cereal recommended for children, contains even more salt (370 mg/oz.). Those who say that these cereals are good because they contain no artificial colors or flavoring overlook the salt. A high salt intake started early in life is more likely to be harmful by causing permanent high blood pressure than is the same high intake started in adulthood.

Remember, all of us could benefit from limiting our salt intake since, over the years, a high intake will help many of us to develop hypertension and heart trouble.

Coffee and Blood Pressure

Some people may be getting treatment for hypertension unnecessarily, the *American Journal of Cardiology* (52:769) warns. This could be the case if their doctors did not know that they had been drinking coffee shortly before their blood pressure was tested.

In a double-blind study comparing the effects of a 250 mg capsule of caffeine (the equivalent of two or three cups of coffee) with those of a placebo, it was found that caffeine raised the blood pressure (BP) significantly. This effect was more marked in people older than 50 than in people younger than 30 and was most powerful in those who were not accustomed to drinking coffee.

The moral of this story is that it would be advisable to abstain from coffee entirely on days when one is to undergo BP testing, especially if one's pressure is near the borderline between normal and levels that are hypertensive.

Alcohol and Blood Pressure

Hypertension that is not responding as well as expected to treatment may suddenly begin to come under control, the *American Family Practitioner* (34#4:182) reports, if the patient takes less alcohol. People usually lose some weight as well when they reduce their alcoholic intake, but this is not the mechanism of the beneficial effect upon hypertension, because the blood pressure usually falls even in those who do not lose any weight

While cutting out alcohol entirely may be necessary for some, at least initially, many find that, by merely drinking substantially less, they can achieve the desired result. We are not discussing alcoholism, for which total abstinence is necessary, but rather, hypertension, in which it may be necessary to cut down from a moderate number of drinks to only a very few.

In fact, between 10 percent and 30 percent of people who have essential hypertension, according to the *Archives of Internal Medicine* (143:29), may be suffering from the effects of too much alcohol, even though they are by no means alcoholics. Merely by drinking socially acceptable amounts of alcohol a few times every day and without ever getting no-ticeably intoxicated, a great number of people get more alcohol than is good for them.

Just five drinks every day (one drink is defined as one can of beer, one and one-fourth ounces (one "shot") of whiskey, one glass of wine, or one cocktail), even if some of them are taken at lunch and others with dinner and in the evening, are more than the average person can tolerate without risk. Small people, of course, would get the same effect from fewer drinks.

The blood pressure elevation caused by "moderate" drink-ing disappears within a few days after the habit is discontin-ued, only to return if the same amount of regular drinking is resumed.

Lest this information about the reversibility of alcohol-induced hypertension be used to justify continuing a poten-tially dangerous habit, it should be understood that the hyper-tension due to taking five or more drinks every day is associ-ated with a much higher than normal incidence of stroke. Stroke, a potential complication of hypertension, regardless of its cause, produces irreversible brain damage, which may even prove fatal. In people who regularly take five or more drinks every day, the Archives reports, there is a three times greater than normal incidence of death from stroke.

In addition, medicines taken to lower the blood pressure (BP), the *Lancet* (1:647) reports, are antagonized by alcoholic drinks. Furthermore, researchers have found, the more alco-hol one takes every day, the greater is this antagonistic effect. Thus the BP of those taking six drinks daily is significantly higher than that of those who drink only two.

If a person significantly reduces his alcohol intake, he may experience a considerable drop in BP, and as a result he will likely feel very tired and weak. Accordingly, those on BP medication who are accustomed to taking several drinks a day will probably need to reduce the dosage should they decide to start drinking less. A doctor's help will be needed in readjusting the dosage so that one can continue to feel comfortable and well.

Cold Remedies and Blood Pressure

Most cold remedies contain two ingredients, an antihistamine to dry up secretions, and a decongestant to shrink blood vessels in the engorged lining of the nose. Although this is a logical combination for most people, it is potentially unsafe for anyone with hypertension (high blood pressure), *American Family Physician* (31#3:183) reports. Understandably, since decongestants shrink swollen nasal membranes by constricting their blood vessels, they can constrict the blood vessels elsewhere in the body as well, particularly when these drugs are taken by mouth.

Because a hypertensive person's vessels are already prone to contract excessively, they react to decongestants with a sustained constriction that raises the blood pressure. According to the *AFP*, this drug-induced hypertension has been sufficiently severe in some cases to cause damage to the heart and strokes from bleeding in the brain. To avoid these dangers, people with hypertension should use cold medications that contain only an antihistamine. In severe cases, when they feel that they cannot do without a decongestant, they should ask their own doctors about taking one in the form of drops or a spray that acts only locally in the nose.

Ginseng and High Blood Pressure

Among 200 normal adults studied at the University of California while taking ginseng daily for long periods, 22 (10 percent) developed hypertension, nervousness, insomnia, rashes, and diarrhea. According to the *Journal of the American Medical Association*, both men and women experienced these side effects in response to the American and foreign varieties of ginseng.

The hypertension was particularly significant in that the average blood pressure of the 22 people involved rose from 125/78 immediately before they started using ginseng to 150/96 13 weeks later. This much hypertension, if continued, is likely to shorten life. Ginseng, taken as tea, capsules, or tablets, is gaining ever wider usage nowadays because many people believe it preserves youth and increases sexual potency. There is no scientific evidence that this is so. Although heavy users may enjoy a feeling of euphoria, the risk of hypertension clearly outweighs the benefits.

Talking and High Blood Pressure

Science 81 (2#6:7) reports that most people's blood pressure becomes elevated while they are talking, even though the subject of their conversation is not causing anger or stress in any way. Researchers at the University of Maryland have seen this happen to 98 percent of the people they have tested. Although the rise is mild in people who have normal blood pressure, the higher the blood pressure to start with, the more it goes up during speech.

Thus, the effect is most pronounced in people who have hypertension. According to the report, this effect of speech is greatly reduced if people talk more slowly and learn to breathe regularly as they converse.

BLOOD PRESSURE— MEASURING

False Blood Pressure Readings

Many elderly people thought to have high blood pressure (BP) may instead have false hypertension, or pseudohypertension, the *American Family Physician* (32#2:242) reports. There are a number of reasons why this could be the case.

One reason that BP readings may be falsely elevated is that the patient has hardening of the arteries. One can find out whether the arteries are hard by feeling the pulse at the wrist while a BP cuff is pumped up on the same arm. If, when the cuff pressure has been raised high enough to obliterate the pulse, the tube-like form of the artery at the wrist can still be felt, this means that it has not collapsed below the inflated cuff and must therefore be abnormally hard. The true BP in such cases can be determined only by inserting a tube directly into the artery through a needle.

Secondly, BP readings may be increased by as much as 10 percent if, while taking them with a stethoscope, one presses the instrument too hard on the arm, the *Western Journal of Medicine* (141:193) reports. To get a true reading it is best to apply the stethoscope with merely a slight pressure. Although increasing the pressure does not alter the systolic BP reading (the upper of the two numbers), the diastolic reading (the lower of the two numbers) can be significantly raised, and it is usually the important one in gauging the effects of anti-hypertension treatment.

Thirdly, blood pressure readings taken with a cuff that is too small for the arm may be as much as 10 mm Hg (millimeters of mercury) too high. This could easily result in a large-armed person taking medicine unnecessarily. According to correspondence in the *New England Journal of Medicine* (306:108), false high readings will not be made if the inflatable bladder in the cuff is long enough (when not inflated) to wrap at least three-fourths of the way round the arm. When a regular adult cuff is too small, a "large adult" or even a "thigh" cuff may be used.

Finally, many people are so nervous while their blood pressure (BP) is being taken in a doctor's office that the readings are abnormally high. This reaction, *Emergency Medicine* (19#11:54) reminds us, often leads to the unwarranted diagnosis of hypertension when, in fact, the BP is perfectly normal. To avoid this problem, the reading could be taken repeatedly, at least five times over a period of five minutes or longer, until it stops falling.

All of these factors can result in people taking BP-lowering medication that they do not need. Not only is this wasteful, but it can make the patient feel light-headed, weak, and tired because, as a result of unnecessary medication, the BP is too low. To avoid this problem, therefore, anyone who is said to be hypertensive should learn to take his or her BPs at home, since one's own readings are much less likely to be misleading.

How to Get Accurate BP Readings

Whenever your blood pressure (BP) is to be taken, whether you are doing it yourself or someone is doing it for you, you should keep several factors in mind so that you can get the most accurate reading.

The *U.S. Pharmacist* (11#7:15) reports that one should rest for at least 15 minutes before a blood pressure reading is taken. This is important because the BP rises to compensate for the increased amount of blood that pools in the legs by gravity as when one is moving about. Without this compensa tory increase of BP, the amount of blood flow to the brain would become inadequate during periods of physical activity. The height of one's BP, furthermore, depends upon how active one has been just before it is taken.

In addition, *Geriatrics* (37#3:38) suggests that whenever possible blood pressure readings be taken with the patient standing. They stress that the decision to change antihypertensive medication dosage should never be based solely upon sitting pressures. This is because when elderly people get up onto their feet, the blood pressure tends to fall, and this drop is especially profound in people taking treatment for hypertension.

Because an abnormal artery in one arm can give misleadingly high blood pressure readings on that side, the pressure should be taken from both arms. The arms, furthermore, should be supported on a table, etc., since a dangling arm gives falsely high blood pressure readings.

Since your BP will also rise if you inhale tobacco smoke or consume caffeine, do not smoke (or even sit near any smokers) or drink coffee, etc., for at least an hour before your pressure is taken.

BLOOD PRESSURE — NATURAL APPROACHES

Calcium for High Blood Pressure

Before giving medications for essential hypertension (high blood pressure which is "spontaneous" rather than secondary to disease of the kidneys or some other organ), the doctor will usually try to help his patient by recommending lifestyle changes, such as weight loss and a restricted salt intake. Usually, only when such measures have been tried for some months and have failed will the doctor prescribe a medication.

Now, *Drug Therapy* (16#11:63) reports, many physicians are also recommending a calcium supplement as part of the lifestyle change. They are doing this because so many of us do not get sufficient calcium to maintain our tissues in good health, and, in some cases, this leads to hypertension. For example, studies at Oregon University revealed that 50 people with hypertension took 22 percent less calcium in their food than did people with normal blood pressure. Also, according to *Medical World News*, epidemiological data strongly suggest that salt causes less hypertension if taken with calcium, too. Since calcium is less expensive and much less likely to cause side effects than blood pressure medications, it is worth trying.

Furthermore, it has been found that by increasing the calcium intake of rats which spontaneously develop hypertension with age, the rise in their blood pressure can largely be prevented.

However, one must not overdo this calcium supplementation since, in excess, it will produce kidney stones, constipation, confusion, vomiting, etc. The safest sources of calcium are low-fat dairy products such as skim milk and cottage cheese, although some dairy products that are good sources of calcium also contain fat and cholesterol, which can lead to atherosclerosis. If you decide to take calcium in tablet form, calcium carbonate is the least expensive and safest product. In any event, never take more than is recommended, and take it in divided doses three times a day rather than all at one time.

Potassium for High Blood Pressure

By strictly limiting their salt intake, people with hypertension can significantly lower their blood pressure. Now, it is realized, potassium intake is also very important. Research reported in the *Lancet* (1:59) has demonstrated a clear relationship between changes in the blood pressure and changes in the amount of potassium intake (when the sodium intake is kept constant). Under these conditions, an increased potassium intake lowers blood pressure, whereas a decreased potassium intake raises it. Best results were obtained in controlling hypertension by both reducing the salt and increasing the potassium in the diet.

Extra potassium can be taken in the form of medicine (e.g., potassium chloride), salt substitutes, or by eating plenty of fruits and vegetables. Orange and apple juice are particularly rich sources. If you are having trouble controlling your blood pressure, taking some extra potassium might make all the difference.

BLOOD PRESSURE— TREATMENT

Is Treatment of High Blood Pressure Really Needed by the Elderly?

Yes, but many people mistakenly believe that some degree of high blood pressure is acceptable as they age. Aiding and abetting them, some physicians used to say that the elderly need a higher than normal blood pressure to force an adequate flow of blood through their hardened and narrowed arteries. These beliefs, unfortunately, are sometimes used to rationalize a do-nothing attitude.

Now, dispelling any doubts about the need for treatment of hypertension in older persons, we have the findings of a study involving several thousand people in Framingham, Mass. who were examined annually for 20 years. The Framingham study, according to *Geriatrics* (35:34), unequivocally links even slightly raised blood pressure to an increased incidence of strokes in the elderly.

On the other side of the coin, *Geriatrics* cautions against excessive lowering of the blood pressure in older people. Although high blood pressure can cause stroke (brain damage) due to bleeding from a burst artery, excessively low blood pressure can do the same thing, but in a different way. When the blood pressure is too low, clots may form in the blood, lodge in an artery, and thereby cut off part of the brain's blood supply.

According to the *Lancet* (1:581), it has been found that hypertensive patients do better if the diastolic BP (the lower of the paired readings) does not come down below 90. While higher than "normal," this seems to be a safer level for people being treated for hypertension. Those whose pressures are brought down below 90, research shows, are less likely to have strokes but have a much greater chance than normal of having coronary heart attacks, especially if they have already had coronary symptoms such as angina (chest pain).

This is understandable because, in such cases, the flow of blood through the heart's coronary arteries is already reduced (by cholesterol deposits). By lowering the BP, we reduce the pumping pressure of the circulation and thus the amount of blood flowing through narrowed arteries as well. So, if you are on a BP medication, tell your doctor if your pressure goes very low, or if you feel unusually tired.

Since dehydration reduces the blood volume and thereby exaggerates the effects of medication that lowers blood pressure, people receiving drugs for hypertension should always take an extra amount of fluid. This is particularly important when fever, sweating, diarrhea, etc., cause increased fluid loss. Also, whenever people taking high blood pressure medication feel faint or dizzy, they should lie down, drink some water, and not get up again until the feeling of faintness goes away. If they do not feel better in a few minutes, medical help should be sought without delay.

According to a review in *Modern Medicine*, the best blood pressure is the lowest one compatible with normal function. This conclusion is based on a study sponsored by the insurance industry which found that "...the untoward effect of blood pressure elevation does not begin at any particular level above the average, but rises progressively with each increase in systolic and diastolic levels recorded. Thus, the life expectancy in patients with below average blood pressure is decidedly better than average."

So, if your blood pressure is 110/70, you stand a better chance of living longer than someone whose pressure is 120/80, everything else being equal, of course.

Side Effects of Diuretics

For more than 30 years, the Thiazide type of diuretics (water pills) have been the most widely used drugs for high blood pressure, but their safety is now in question. According to *Geriatrics* (39#1:40), there is a side effect of diuretics that can happen so gradually that it can quite easily be overlooked. By excessively reducing the body's salt and water content, these medicines may also be reducing the blood volume so much that the blood pressure sinks dangerously low. Persons with extreme salt and water loss are likely to experience weakness, giddiness, and confusion, and may even faint and fall down, injuring themselves, when they suddenly try to stand. This effect, however, can be reversed by reducing the dose or giving some extra salt.

More recently, it has been discovered that some people taking a thiazide develop heartbeat irregularities, some of which are serious or even fatal. This risk, too, according to *Drug Therapy* (18#8:49), can be eliminated if the doctor gives some extra potassium and magnesium by mouth to prevent drug-induced depletion of these minerals from the body.

Most recently, thiazides have been found to increase cholesterol levels. Even worse, perhaps, is their effect on the "bad" LDL type of cholesterol, which increases by an average of 10 percent. Since no way of reversing this undesirable effect has been discovered, many doctors now use other diuretics instead.

Anyone whose cholesterol level is usually in the 150-180 mg range probably need not worry. But, for those with levels above normal, thiazide medication probably should be replaced.

However, a high blood pressure that rises out of control because of discontinued medication is more immediately dangerous than a high cholesterol level. One should therefore never discontinue or alter the dosage of a thiazide without the prescribing physician's consent.

Actually, anyone who is taking a diuretic ought to monitor his blood pressure at home, taking his own readings or getting someone to do it for him. The doctor should be asked ahead of time about the lowest level that is safe, and, if the pressure falls below that, he should be told about it right away.

Side Effects of Other Blood Pressure Treatments

Other than diuretic drugs (discussed above), most drugs used in hypertension work by relaxing the muscular walls of the blood vessels and are more likely to cause side effects because they relax other muscles, too. For example, they can cause difficulty in passing urine (due to relaxation of the bladder muscle), constipation (by relaxing the intestinal muscles), and sometimes impotence in men.

Even without drug treatment, many people feel dizzy momentarily after suddenly standing up. Called postural hypotension, this occurs when, for a few moments, blood pools in the veins of the legs and does not get up to the brain. Blood vessels slackened by drugs are more likely to cause this effect, and patients taking multiple blood pressure medications may have severe postural hypotension and even lose consciousness if they stand up too quickly or stand still for too long (movement assists the circulation).

Whenever people on blood pressure drugs feel dizzy, they should immediately stretch and yawn and move their legs to boost the circulation. Hypertensive patients liable to dizziness under these conditions should never shut themselves in a telephone booth, because being held upright after fainting could be fatal. The combined effects of blood pooling in the legs and continuing to remain propped upright prevents a life-sustaining blood supply reaching up to the brain. Falling, although it may cause injury, instantly lowers the head so that blood can flow into it by gravity.

If side effects become a frequent problem, the situation can be corrected by changing the dosage or by switching drugs. This needs to be done under medical supervision. Whatever happens, hypertensive patients must continue taking some medications regularly every day because, without it, their lives will be shortened.

BLOOD PRESSURE — WARNING SIGNS

A Newly Recognized Cause of Suddenly Worsening Hypertension

Hypertension tends to progress with age, but usually does so gradually. Suddenly worsening hypertension, according to *Modern Medicine* (50#2:276), can, among other things, be caused by mood-elevating drugs that are used in the treatment of mental depression.

Even though these medications do not usually raise the blood pressure in otherwise healthy persons, existing hypertension tends to be worsened by them and may rise rapidly out of control. To avoid this problem, hypertensive persons taking anti-depressant medication should monitor the blood pressure more closely than usual, and, if necessary, take extra anti-hypertensive medication.

Nosebleeds

In adults, nosebleeds are much more likely to be symptomatic of serious conditions than they are in children. Apart from lesions in the nose, conditions such as overdosage with certain drugs (e.g: blood thinners such as Dicumarol), diabetes, blood disorders, and kidney failure must be looked for in a careful medical examination. One of the most common causes of nosebleeds in adults is hypertension, or high blood pressure (BP).

Since anyone who has just lost a lot of blood could be in shock, and thereby have a lower BP than usual, the *Journal of Laryngology and Otology* (98:277) recommends that the BP be taken several times after the patient has fully recovered. In this way, cases of hypertension that have been responsible for nosebleeding will not be missed.

Special Risk in Hypertension Newly Defined

Fever not only makes sick persons flushed and sweaty, but it can markedly lower their blood pressure too. This, no doubt, helps to account for the weakness and lightheadedness which usually accompany fever. Not recognized until now, this fall in the blood pressure adds to the effect of medicines that lower blood pressure and thereby poses a special risk for people with hypertension.

According to a report in the *New England Journal of Medicine* (302:865), a patient who had regularly been taking two antihypertensive drugs developed a cold with fever and became so weak that he was unable to get up and walk without extreme faintness and staggering. At that time, his blood pressure was found to be excessively low. Not bothered by this any more after the fever went away, he again experienced this problem the next night when the fever returned.

Sudden reductions in blood pressure of this kind could result in bone-breaking falls or bring on strokes or heart attacks. Accordingly, people taking medicines for hypertension should not get out of bed when they are suffering from fever unless there is someone in attendance.

BREATHING PROBLEMS

Illness Due to Stuffy Homes

In tightly built homes that minimize air leakage too efficiently, occupants complain of many symptoms, including breathlessness, headache, nasal stuffiness, eye irritation, coughing, frequent colds, sore throats, rashes, weakness, and insomnia. So troublesome are these complaints that many people have abandoned their new homes.

A mystery at first, the symptoms are now known to be due to the accumulation of formaldehyde vapor and other toxic gases in the home. In less tightly constructed houses, a greater exchange of air with the outdoors prevents this accumulation.

The most common source of formaldehyde in older homes is the urea-formaldehyde foam sprayed into attics and hollow walls to improve their insulation. This material should not be confused with the harmless light weight sheets of polyurethane and polystyrene foam currently being used for insulation in the newest homes. Unlike urea-formaldehyde foam, these solid products are "cured" before use and do not give off toxic fumes unless set on fire. Even though urea-formaldehyde foam is not used in new houses, a small amount of formaldehyde seeps into them from particle board and plywood, both of which are made with formaldehyde-containing glue.

When homes are very tightly sealed, according to the *Journal of the American Medical Association* (245:267), we should also be concerned about volatile solvents from paint and hair sprays, carbon monoxide from wood burning stoves, and ozone from electrostatic air filters, hair dryers, and toasters. By opening some windows for a few minutes every day, you can prevent accumulation of these substances in your home.

Saline Drops for Nasal Obstructions

When an allergy or a head cold thickens the lining membranes of the nose and fills it with an excess of mucus, nasal breathing becomes almost impossible. In such cases, many people find it helpful to use nose drops made from table salt and warm water. This liquid is put into one nostril at a time (while the other is pressed closed) and sniffed repeatedly until it comes through to the back of the throat. It should then be spat out rather than swallowed.

The latest news on this topic, according to *Pediatric Alert* (5:10), is that, if the salt solution is too strong, it will irritate the nose and make matters worse. The correct strength is achieved by adding only one-fourth of a teaspoonful of salt to eight ounces (a large drinking glassful) of warm water. Most people tend to make it too strong.

Medication Strengthens Breathing

Those who become permanently short of breath because of chronic bronchitis and lung damage after decades of heavy smoking have what it called chronic obstructive pulmonary disease (COPD). Ultimately, they become blue in the face (when the lungs no longer allow the blood to obtain all of the body's oxygen needs) and develop heart failure. Fatigue and weakness then develop in the overworked muscles of the chest making matters even worse.

In searching for ways to strengthen breathing and counter-act the respiratory muscle fatigue, physicians have discovered that theophylline, the time-honored medication for asthma, has a consistently useful effect, the *New England Journal of Medicine* (311:349) reports.

Taken twice daily in doses of 500 mg for one week, theophylline improves the strength of the diaphragm and the efficiency of respiration. This effect is enough to cause marked improvement in COPD patients and is maintained for at least three weeks, even after the drug is discontinued.

How often theophylline courses need to be repeated remains to be established. Theophylline, incidentally, is an ingredient of coffee and tea, which also contain the closely related chemical, caffeine. It, too, improves the efficiency of respiration and the strength of the muscles, including the diaphragm.

Aspirin and the Nose

The effect of aspirin on the lining of the nose, surprisingly, is not advantageous, the *British Medical Journal* (290:1171) reports. Aspirin, it has been discovered by precise scientific measurements, reduces air flow through the nasal passages, an effect brought about by congestion and swelling of the nasal mucous membranes.

The importance of this story is clear: if you are suffering from a cold and experience some difficulty in breathing through the nose, aspirin is liable to make matters worse. It was interesting to note that, in the same study and under exactly the same conditions, vitamin C had no bad effect upon the air flow through the nose.

A Reliable Treatment for Snoring

Snoring may result whenever the upper airway is narrowed. It can therefore occur in a variety of conditions, including the common cold, allergy, nasal septum deviation, enlarged tonsils, adenoids, etc.

Most snorers, however, have no narrowing of the upper airway while awake and only begin to do so as they fall asleep. It is then that the tongue relaxes, slides backwards and downwards and, in snorers, almost blocks the throat. Passing through these "narrows," breathed air vibrates and forms the characteristic sounds.

In such tongue-swallowing cases, according to the *Journal of the American Medical Association* (244:1783), snoring can be prevented if the snorer wears a foam rubber neck-bracing collar while in bed. By holding the chin up, the collar prevents the tongue, which is attached to the chin, from sliding backwards far enough to block the throat. The collars are available at most drug stores.

Sinusitis and Antihistamines

Even though sinusitis is associated with congestion and excessive mucus, treatment with medications that dry the nose is not really helpful, *Drug Therapy* (16#7:132) reports. In fact, antihistamines and decongestants can make matters worse. They shrink the mucous membrane lining of the nose and sinuses by constricting its blood vessels and thus drastically reduce its blood flow in the process.

If an antibiotic is being taken to deal with the bacterial cause of the sinusitis, little of it will gain access to the sinus when its blood supply has been reduced in this way, since antibiotics depend upon the bloodstream for their transportation in the tissues. Furthermore, antihistamines and decongestants slow the beat of the cilia (minute tail-like processes on the cells at the surface of the mucous membranes), the repeated wave-like movements of which sweep dust, mucus, and bacteria up and out from the body.

Thus, when sinusitis does not resolve by itself, a physician will usually be able to cure it with antibiotics alone. Should that fail, he may have to drain the infected sinus. Do not try to treat it yourself with an antihistamine or a decongestant, since these drugs are likely to do more harm than good.

Crash Helmet Hazard

Crash helmets with plastic visors can dangerously diminish the wearer's oxygen supply, especially when worn together with a scarf, ski mask, or any other garment that restricts air flow around the chin and neck. According to the *British Medical Journal* (284:774), crash helmet design was pioneered by neurosurgeons whose major preoccupation was in preventing brain trauma.

So little attention has been paid to venting helmets that blood levels of oxygen and carbon dioxide (the waste gas) can easily become abnormal. Oxygen deprivation has an intoxicating effect that could well account for many accidents, particularly in cold weather when helmeted drivers bundle up against the cold.

CANCER— CAUSES AND LINKS

Talc's Danger Recognized

Most of the talc produced before 1972, *Cutis* (37:328) reports, was contaminated with some asbestos, which is not surprising since both of these substances are crystalline forms of magnesium silicate and often found side by side in the same mine.

Talc miners, like asbestos miners, have a higher than normal share of health problems, often develop scarring of the lungs, and have a three to four times normal incidence of lung cancer. Exposure to asbestos dust in the workplace often results in tumors in the chest and lungs as many as 20-30 years later.

It was hoped that cleaning up talc by removing its asbestos component would reduce the incidence of cancer, especially cancer of the lung, that had been associated with the use of both asbestos and talc products. Now, however, it has been discovered that women who employ talcum regularly as a part of their feminine hygiene routine are three times more likely than normal to develop cancer of the ovary. Talc has been found deeply embedded in the ovaries by traveling up the vagina and then through the uterus and Fallopian tubes.

Talc-containing powder is also often applied to babies' bottoms whenever their diapers are changed. However, Pediatric Notes (9:106) reports, doctors are becoming increasingly wary of recommending these powders for the skin care of infants. Even when a talcum powder is guaranteed asbestos-free, it is safer to avoid it since one can never be sure of the other ingredients, and it is not a good idea for babies to be breathing dust, even if it is asbestos-free.

Because of the potential cancer risk, many doctors are now urging their patients to stop dusting themselves and their children with talcum powder.

Cancer and the Pill

Two very important articles about research with oral contraceptives were published right next to each other in a recent issue of the *Lancet* (2:926).

The first of these provided convincing data to show that breast cancer is more common than usual, significantly so, in young women who have regularly taken an oral contraceptive (OC) for many years. After reviewing the histories of 314 cases of breast cancer in women under the age of 37 years who had been treated at the University of California in Los Angeles (UCLA) medical school, researchers found that the incidence of these tumors was four times higher than normal among those women who had used an OC for at least six years before they had reached the age of 25.

In addition, the researchers discovered, the OCs that were the most dangerous in this regard were those containing relatively large amounts of the synthetic hormones known as progestogens. While all OCs need to contain about the same amount of an estrogen of some sort to make them effective in preventing pregnancy, their progestogen content, which is less essential and which controls the timing, amount, and duration of the cyclic menstrual bleeding, varies rather considerably in amount in the different brands. It is the progestogenic component of OCs that increases a woman's chances of developing breast cancer, the UCLA researchers believe.

Brands of oral contraceptive that are of relatively "high potency" so far as their progestogen content is concerned include Demulen, Enovid 5, Enovid 10, Lo/Ovral, Ortho-Novum 10, Ovral, Ovulen, Norinyl 10, and Norlestin 2.5.

If what the UCLA researchers have said is correct, it would be safer for women who are using any one of these OCs to switch to another brand. Furthermore, this report should also serve to motivate women who have used OCs to carefully examine their breasts every month, regularly and without fail. Local chapters of the American Cancer Society (see your telephone book) provide an excellent booklet on how to do this properly. Early detection of breast tumors makes them much more curable and greatly helps the surgeon in restoring the appearance of the breasts to normal.

The same issue of the *Lancet* (2:930) contained further bad news about oral contraceptives. Several times already, it has been suggested that uterine cervix cancer is more common than usual among long-term users of OCs, but there has been a reluctance to blame the pill for this since other factors (such as age, number of pregnancies, etc.) also undoubtedly influence the situation.

Now, the *Lancet* reports, there is at last some more definite evidence to implicate OCs as one of the contributing factors. Oxford University (England) medical school gynecologists have shown that cervical cancer is at least 2.2 times more common in women who have used OCs than it is in women of the same age and number of pregnancies, etc., who have used an IUD for contraception instead.

Again, we must emphasize that early cancer detection saves lives. For this reason, any woman who has taken an OC should get herself examined and have a PAP smear regularly in accordance with her doctor's instructions.

Smoking and Cancer

There is now good evidence to show that smokers' lung cancer is due to radioactivity carried down into the lungs with smoke. Radioactive lead contained in tobacco is volatilized by the heat of burning and condenses onto the membranous lining of the airways, especially where the passages divide (bifurcations). Over the years, more and more radioactive lead (which "decays" into radioactive polonium) accumulates. Whether or not it stays at these sites largely depends upon how normal a person's lungs remain.

If damaged beyond repair by tar and infection, the membrane's lining cells lose their cilia (tail-like processes that, by constantly beating, waft inhaled particles up and out of the chest) and become unable to rid themselves of the radioactive contamination.

Eight groups of scientists recently wrote about this to *New England Journal of Medicine*, which published their letters together in the same issue (307:309). Most significantly, they reported, discovery of radioactive lead in smoke has been the most powerful anti-smoking influence they had ever encountered. News of it, apparently, has convinced many heavy smokers, for the first time, to stop smoking immediately.

It has also been found that the cancer-producing effect of smoking may not all be due to damage done directly to the lungs. According to the *Medical Journal of Australia* (2:425), the lymphocytes (one of the many types of white blood cell that defend the body against invading microorganisms) in smokers become much more sluggish than usual.

In particular, the ability of the lymphocytes to become "killer cells," which attack any other cells of the body that begin to behave abnormally (e.g: become cancerous), is greatly reduced by smoking. This could explain why smokers have so many more infections than non-smokers, and why their tumors, such as melanomas, grow and spread more quickly to other parts of the body. Because the lymphocytes quickly regain their normal killer cell activities when smoking is stopped, it is never too late to give up the habit.

Environmental Factors and Colon Cancer

Cancers of the large intestine (the colon and rectum) are most common among people who live far from the equator and rare among those who live close to it. Rare in Africa, Asia, and Japan, colorectal cancer kills 45,000 people a year in the United States. Since immigrants from low-risk countries acquire America's high incidence of colorectal cancer, environmental rather than genetic factors must be at work. This geographic variation, it is now understood, is linked to two factors: the amount of sunlight to which people are exposed and the diet they are accustomed to eating.

How does sunlight relate to cancer of the colon? Since sunlight increases the skin's production of vitamin D, and this vitamin improves calcium absorption, people in the tropics rarely suffer from calcium deficiency (if there is no famine), a problem common in those farther north or south. Calcium, the *New England Journal of Medicine* (313:1413) reports, protects the colon and rectum from the irritating and cancer-promoting effects of bile acids by precipitating and thus inactivating them

Members of families prone to colorectal cancer, the *Lancet* (1:307) reports, have intestinal lining cells that are often replaced by new cells and are unusually sensitive to bile acid irritation. This high replacement rate and irritability, it has just been shown, can be reduced to normal by supplementing the diet with extra calcium and vitamin D. Thus, by supplementing our diets with one gram of calcium and 400 units of vitamin D every day, we can greatly reduce the risk of colorectal cancer.

Dietary fiber is another factor which relates to colon cancer. A carcinogen (a substance that transforms normal tissue into cancer) has recently been discovered in the feces of Americans, but there is little if any of it in Africans, Asians, or Japanese. The substance is formed from bile by bacteria in the intestines. Acidity, according to the *Lancet* (1:1081), inhibits reproduction of these carcinogen-producing bacteria. This may explain why Africans, Asiatics, and Japanese rarely have colorectal cancer. Their high fiber diet probably protects them because fibers are digested down into acids. Also, a high fiber diet has an ability to speed the passage of all substances (including carcinogens and promoters of cancer growth) through the intestines, thereby minimizing their contact with

94

the intestinal wall and reducing their cancer-producing effects.

Fitting neatly with this theory is the fact that bile is produced most plentifully by people who eat a lot of animal fat. To protect ourselves, therefore, we should eat less animal fat and much more fruit and vegetables. Every day, we should also take a few tablespoonfuls of bran.

See also the article, "Is There a Relationship Between Cancer and Cholesterol?" on page 96.

Hepatitis and Liver Cancer— the Link

Liver cancer, relatively rare in North American and Europe, is mankind's most common tumor in the tropics. There, also, infectious hepatitis is much more common. Research reported in the *Lancet* (2:1394) suggests that Hepatitis-B virus (HBV), known to be responsible for many cases of infectious hepatitis, may also cause cancer of the liver.

Every virus has its characteristic sequence of nucleic acids in the chemical known as DNA. Like a fingerprint, HBV's sequence is detectable in the blood and liver during acute infectious hepatitis but, after recovery, it usually disappears. It is only people whose tissues continue harboring HBV who, years later, develop cancer of the liver. Significantly, by the time they develop liver cancer, the HBV pattern has blended with their own DNA pattern, forming a hybrid, especially in the tissues of the tumor.

Consistent with these facts is the observation that liver cancer, although rare in animals, is the most frequent cause of death in woodchucks at the Philadelphia Zoo. The woodchuck is one of the few creatures, other than man, to be made ill by a virus with the nucleic acid sequence of HBV.

Since infection with HBV increases our liability to liver

cancer about 20-fold, all victims of active hepatitis should be isolated and their contacts given immune globulin.

Dust and Cancer of the Nose

A 300 to 400-fold increased risk of nasal cancer was discovered at the turn of the century among workers engaged in nickel production. This was eventually attributed to dust from the ore.

Now, the same sort of problem has come to light among people engaged in furniture making, especially in the United States. These nasal cancers, reports the *Lancet* (1:856), appear to be due to hardwood dust. Canadian furniture makers, in contrast, do not have a higher than usual incidence of nasal cancer. However, they work with softwood rather than hardwood.

Another group of workers with nasal cancer due to dust are the shoe makers and those in the shoe repair industry. Chemicals used in tanning leather rather than the leather itself, it is believed, cause these tumors.

Since we may have to wait many years to discover whether or not the dust produced in a new industry is going to produce cancers of the respiratory tract (cancer of the lung is known to be caused by other types of dust), it would be safer for all workers who are exposed to dust of any sort to wear a mask. See the related article, "Talc's Danger Recognized" on page 89.

Is There a Relationship Between Cancer and Cholesterol?

Just about everybody knows that the more cholesterol you

have in your blood, the more likely you are to die from a heart attack. This association, confirmed over and over again in many parts of the world, is why most physicians now advise people to avoid foods rich in cholesterol and, if necessary, to take medicine to lower the blood cholesterol. But is there also a link between cholesterol levels and cancer?

One surprising opinion was recently reported in the *Lancet* (2:603) by a University of Minnesota researcher. He said that, after studying the medical histories of 284 professional men in Minneapolis and St. Paul, he had found more deaths from cancer than expected among men who had reduced their blood cholesterol levels by dieting, etc. He even went so far as to suggest that high blood cholesterol levels may help to protect the body against cancer. It must also be stated, though, that not everyone who analyzed the Minneapolis-St. Paul data agreed with him about this.

So important is this issue that the government recently appointed a team of experts from the National Heart Institute and the National Cancer Institute to examine it from every angle. According to the *Wall Street Journal*, the experts concluded, "...the two institutes agree that the risk of heart disease from high cholesterol levels seems to exceed the small and uncertain risk of cancer from low cholesterol levels. Therefore, it is still prudent for anyone with high cholesterol levels to attempt to lower them."

Researchers at Chicago's Northwestern Medical School go much farther. They suspect that it is the excess cholesterol in the American diet that accounts for our high incidence of colon carcinoma. They reached this conclusion after studying the colon cancer death rates of different countries in relation to their diets. (See also the article, "Environmental Factors and Colon Cancer." on page 93.)

Finland is an exception to the rule that high fat intake is linked with high death rates from heart attack and carcinoma of the colon. The Finnish diet, which provides the world's highest fat intake, is associated with the world's highest heart attack rate. Surprisingly, however, Finland has one of the world's lowest colon cancer death rates.

Looking into this more closely, Northwestern researchers found that the Finnish diet is an unusual one. Finns eat excessive amount of butter and cream but very little fat from meat or eggs. Thus, their high fat intake consists mostly of triglycerides but contains relatively little cholesterol. The Northwestern study therefore suggests that cholesterol plays a far more important role in colon cancer than do any other types of fat.

Although probably not a carcinogen (a cause of cancer), they think cholesterol is a "promoter" (a substance which multiplies the effect of carcinogens). Diets rich in cholesterol would thus enhance the probability of colon cancer, especially in families that are naturally more than usually prone to develop that type of tumor.

So, if you wish to minimize your chances of getting cancer of the colon, use eggs sparingly, trim the fat off your meat, and take enough bran every day (most people need two to three heaped tablespoonfuls) to make your bowels move easily.

Power Lines and Leukemia

Does exposure to the strong electrical and magnetic field surrounding high voltage power cables cause cancer or leukemia? Experts on this subject differ, but, according to recent letters to the editor of the *Lancet* (2:1160), the incidence of leukemia among some types of electrical workers in Los

Angeles during the eight-year period 1972-79 was higher than expected.

Men who climbed the poles and worked closest to high tension cables (both electric power and telephone linemen), the records show, were five to eight times more likely to develop acute myelogenous leukemia than were members of the general population. This difference was statistically significant. Smaller increases in acute leukemia incidence (two to five times the normal) were seen in power station operators, motion picture projectionists, arc welders, and electrical engineers.

Even though leukemia is more common than normal in those who work near high voltage power lines, experts remain undecided about the danger of those weaker electromagnetic fields to which we are all exposed. Nevertheless, the *Boston Globe* reports, millions are being spent to investigate this matter, and, in the absence of proof that it is safe to do so, it is prudent not to live close to high voltage power lines.

If there is any danger of leukemia from this source, it would apply especially to pregnant women and children. Possibly, too, we should avoid the magnetic fields of electric blankets. However, since they are so useful when it is cold, we can compromise by putting them on in the evening and unplugging them just before getting into bed.

Diesel Engine Fumes

Railroad employees whose occupation exposes them to diesel engine fumes, according to *Medical World News* (23#9:22), have a lung cancer rate almost 40 percent higher than that of other railroad workers. This is consistent with the well-established fact that diesel exhaust soot is rich in hydrocarbon pollutants that are known to be highly carcinogenic for animals. Harvard researchers who made this survey agreed with railroad officials that their findings are preliminary, and that their study was too small to establish cause-and-effect.

Nevertheless, because diesel-powered vehicles produce so much black smoke, we urge readers who spend much time driving near trucks and buses to keep their windows up, at least until they are out of heavy traffic.

Drinking Water — a New Cause of Cancer?

A study carried out by the President's Council of Environmental Quality and reported in *Science* (211:694) suggests an association between three common types of cancer (rectum, colon, and bladder) and chlorinated water. This carcinogenic effect is not thought to be caused by chlorine itself but, rather, by cancer-producing chemicals formed by the action of chlorine on organic substances naturally present in surface water. Well water, unlike surface water, lacks these substances and, according to *Science*, is therefore not associated with an increased incidence of cancer, even if chlorinated.

How can we avoid cancer if even water is not safe? We should not be too alarmed, *Science* suggests, because chlorinated water probably does not even double the "normal" rate of cancer and risks less than two-fold are generally subject to doubt. Regardless of this comforting thought, federal regulations require that chlorine compounds in our water be kept below one part per 10 million. Meanwhile, remember that the chlorine in our water kills bacteria, thereby protecting us from dangerous epidemics, a benefit which clearly outweighs this newly-defined potential and marginal risk of cancer.

Does Barbecued Food Cause Cancer?

There is no evidence that we significantly increase our risks of getting cancer by eating barbecued food, according to an expert who answered this question in the *British Medical Journal* (292:182). Furthermore, he states, this question is really out of date in that it indicates a lack of understanding that there are literally thousands of substances that could help to cause cancer, together with those that can prevent it, in everything we eat, and that in this regard barbecued food does not differ very much from food prepared in other ways.

Whether or not we develop cancer as a result of the things we eat, therefore, depends on much more than merely the presence or absence of barbecued food in our diet. If you like barbecued food, then, you can relax and enjoy it.

Salads — Life Threatening for Some?

Uncooked vegetables, including lettuce, onions, carrots, cucumbers, tomatoes, radishes, etc., naturally harbor a great number of bacteria that are ordinarily harmless but that may become the source of potentially fatal infections for very sick patients taking antibiotics. Billions of bacteria inhabiting the intestines of healthy persons usually compete so successfully for nourishment with bacteria carried down with food that the latter rapidly die out.

In the large doses commonly given to very sick patients in hospital, antibiotics destroy so many of the body's normal bacteria that food-borne bacteria gain a foothold in the intestines, multiply, and then migrate to other parts of the body to set up pneumonia, septicemia (blood poisoning), etc.

For this reason, cancer specialists writing in the *New England Journal of Medicine* (304:443) urge that very sick persons under the influence of antibiotics, especially cancer patients whose immunity is already impaired, should not be given salads and should eat only food which has been completely sterilized.

CANCER— EARLY WARNING

Leg Ulcers

People with varicose veins, diabetes, or hardening of the arteries often must learn to accept an unhealed leg ulcer as the inevitable complication of poor circulation. While it is true that skin healing can be greatly impaired by these conditions, it is also true that leg ulcers due to poor circulation ought to improve when given appropriate treatment.

A report in the *British Medical Journal* (286:207) tells of patients with long-standing varicose veins or diabetes who also had ulcerated skin of the lower leg that stubbornly failed to heal for periods of up to 10 years. Skin cancer, although not obvious, was ultimately found to be the underlying fault in all. The moral of this story is that, regardless of the status of the circulation, one must always suspect skin cancer and have appropriate tests performed when a leg ulcer fails to show any signs of healing after four months of medical treatment.

Pigmented Moles

Irregularly shaped pigmented moles that appear on the skin at any time after birth, medically known as dysplastic nevi, and which are over six mm (about a quarter of an inch) in diameter, are likely to grow and turn into melanomas (a type of skin cancer) at some time before one is 70 years old, the journal *Cutis* (34#5:498) reports. Accordingly, one should examine large moles regularly every month and, if there is any doubt, measure them to make sure that they are not growing. In addition, these moles should be examined by a physician every six months. Any that are getting bigger should be removed before they can become melanomas.

Delay in Diagnosis of Testicular Tumors Costs Lives

Monthly self-examination of the breasts by women is generally acknowledged to be an efficient way of detecting tumors while they are still likely to be curable. Why then don't men take the same trouble in detecting testicular tumors? The answer, of course, is that testicular tumors are much less common than tumors of the breast.

Nevertheless, according to the *Southern Medical Journal* (78:33), men all too frequently procrastinate after finding a mass in the scrotum. When diagnosis and surgical treatment are carried out early and before a testicular tumor has spread beyond the scrotum, cure can be obtained in over 90 percent of cases. Three months seems to be a critical period. When men delay longer than this before seeking help, their tumors are more likely to have spread, and survival then drops to less than 50 percent.

Unfortunately, the man who discovers an abnormal testicular mass tends to find an excuse for not doing anything about it. Such masses are usually painless, and this suggests to non-medical people that they can't really be dangerous. Nothing could be more misleading, because the majority of testicular tumors are highly malignant. For this reason, *Emergency Medicine* (12#17:167) recommends that, using both hands, all men should systematically feel the contents of the scrotum every month and report to a physician immediately if they detect anything abnormal. Taking only a minute, this procedure can save many lives.

CANCER—PREVENTION AND TREATMENT

Vitamin A at Last Proven to Protect Against Cancer

Vitamin A deficiency is a well known cause of increased susceptibility to cancer in laboratory animals. It also allows cultures of normal cells growing in test tubes to become more easily transformed into cancer cells by carcinogenic chemicals or by radiation. Applying this knowledge to research in human cancer, physicians long ago measured the blood levels of vitamin A in people with cancer and found them to be lower than those in people of the same age and race, etc., who did not have cancer.

Although this finding has been confirmed in several

human studies, critics have argued that this does not prove a cause-and-effect relationship. Cancer, they have suggested, may use up extra amounts of vitamin A and thus be the cause rather than the result of low vitamin A blood levels.

Settling this dispute once and for all, cancer researchers have at last clearly established that low vitamin A blood levels in otherwise healthy persons more than doubles their chances of developing cancer in the next five years. This is consistent with a Norwegian study in which it was found that men classified as having a low vitamin A intake were four times more prone to develop lung cancer than equally heavy smokers taking a normal amount of vitamin A. There are, of course, other factors at work in causing cancer.

The message is clear: Make sure that you take the proper amount of vitamin A every day. One daily multi-vitamin tablet containing 10,000 units (or three milligrams) of vitamin A should be enough. Only pregnant women need more than this. Excess vitamin A is to be avoided because it can cause joint pains, hair loss, yellowness and dryness of the skin, and liver disease.

A New Boost for Cancer Immunotherapy

The National Cancer Institute has launched a large scale (200 patients) test of an immune hormone called thymosin that could make non-surgical cancer therapy more successful. Cancer specialists are investigating thymosin's possible role in immunotherapy, the process of stimulating the body's own defenses against the disease.

Many authorities believe that cancer cells gain a foothold when our immune system becomes less efficient in seeking them out and destroying them. Unfortunately, this immune function is largely under the control of the thymus glands, two soft, pinkish gray lobes found in the upper chest that gradually disappear as we age.

The body employs chemical messengers like thymosin to alert various components of the immune system to their roles. According to a report in *Science 81* (2:73), when thymosin levels are artificially increased, the immune system reacts by fighting cancer cells with greater vigor.

One study of 55 patients with a particularly difficult-to-treat cancer, small cell cancer of the lung, was summarized. Among 21 patients who received the highest doses of the drug, six were alive and free of disease after two years. Average survival time in this group increased from 240 to 450 days. While no firm conclusion can be reached from such a small study, larger studies now in progress should demonstrate whether a deficient immune defense system against cancer can always be corrected by thymosin, and for how long the effect lasts.

Coffee Enemas for Cancer?

Although MDs deplore the fact that some cancer victims try naturopathic diets first, thereby postponing and reducing their chances of responding to conventional treatment, most physicians believe that dietary treatment is otherwise intrinsically harmless.

This, however, cannot be said of a bizarre naturopathic cancer treatment which is being practiced just south of the Mexican border. The regimen consists of natural foods, minerals, vitamins, iodine, and thyroid extract given by mouth, as well as coffee, given rectally in enemas about every two hours. Autopsy studies, according to the *Journal of the American Medical Association* (244:1608), have shown that at least two deaths have been actually caused by the coffee enemas rather than by the tumors for which they were given.

Even conventional medical treatments for cancer, it could be argued, are potentially dangerous and, in some cases, have produced fatal complications. While this is true, conventional medical treatments, unlike coffee enemas, do have well established track records of having prolonged life and even curing many patients of cancer at just about every hospital around the world. That, unfortunately, cannot be said of coffee enemas.

Prostate Cancer Treatment

Enlargement of the prostate, whether due to cancer or to the benign swelling that occurs so commonly in aging men has, until recently, been most often treated by the operation in which pieces of tissue are removed with an instrument that is passed up the urethra, the urinary passage in the penis. Called transurethral resection (TUR), this is easier than surgically removing the entire prostate through the lower abdomen, an operation known as prostatectomy. Furthermore, until now, TUR was much less likely than prostatectomy to cause impotence because it does not injure nerves supplying the penis. Prostatectomy, as usually performed, did injure those nerves, thereby often causing permanent impotence. Understandably then, even though cure of prostate cancer is less likely with TUR than with prostatectomy, TUR has been the more popular procedure.

Now, thanks to a new type of prostatectomy operation that has just recently been developed at Johns Hopkins Hospital and reported in *Prostate* (4:473), we can at last have the best of both worlds.

Because it spares the nerves of the penis, this new operation is most unlikely to cause lasting impotence. (For some weeks or months after prostate surgery of any kind, it must be understood, all men will experience at least some degree of impotence). Another advantage of the new prostatectomy surgery, which is performed through the lower abdomen, is the completeness with which it removes all tumor tissue. With these positive features, it is likely to become the treatment of choice.

CHILD SAFETY

Overheating and Crib Death

Until now, the cause of crib death (also known as the Sudden Infant Death Syndrome) has remained a mystery, although, in many cases, it has been noted that the deceased infant had an infection (usually a "cold") for a day or so before its untimely end. Research published in the *Lancet* (2:1199) offers a new and plausible explanation for this unexpected kind of death which acknowledges infection but does not give it all the blame.

In short, overheating has been proposed as the immediate cause of these deaths. Analysis of a large number of crib deaths has revealed a number of reasons for overheating, including fever due to an infection, too much clothing or too many blankets on the infant, and too high a temperature in the room. More than one of these causes coexisted in many cases.

Overheating is known to cause convulsions (febrile

seizures), which generate extra body heat as well, thus constituting a vicious circle. Furthermore, apnea, a lack of breathing that (if prolonged) can be fatal, always accompanies convulsions. In newly born infants, apnea may even occur instead of convulsions.

So, if overheating is truly the main cause of crib death, and in the absence of a better explanation, one should avoid overdressing or covering a baby with too many blankets or keeping the house too warm, especially if the baby has an infection.

Swimming Infants

Even though babies can learn to swim quite well during their first year of life and may be relatively safe from drowning, there is a danger of water intoxication if one does not supervise them carefully when they are in the water. *Pediatrics* (70:599) reports the case of a 10-month-old boy who, during a swimming lesson, swallowed nearly 10 percent of his body weight in water and, an hour later, became drowsy and had convulsive seizures.

Water intoxication, cautions *Pediatrics*, urgently needs treatment with intravenous injections of a special concentrated saline to "thicken" the blood, and quickly becomes life-threatening if overlooked and left untreated. So, if your children or grandchildren learn to swim when they are very small, watch them closely all the time they are in the water to make sure that they do not drink it.

CHOLESTEROL

What Is a "High" Cholesterol Blood Level?

Unquestionably, those with a high blood level of cholesterol are, in general, much more likely than others to have a coronary heart attack or stroke. Cholesterol settles out onto the walls of their arteries and narrows them, so that they easily become completely blocked. Accordingly, *Circulation* (72:686) recommends, those who have high cholesterol should be treated to bring it down to a safer level. The big question, of course, is what is meant by "high cholesterol."

In answering this, we must first explain that cholesterol is a mixture of HDL (high density lipoprotein) and LDL (low density lipoprotein), and that HDL is good and LDL is bad. One needs to worry about a cholesterol level only if the LDL fraction is present in excess.

This said, we can go on to say that anyone with a cholesterol above 230 mg-percent needs to be on a strict low-cholesterol diet, and that if the cholesterol is 260 mg-percent or more, a cholesterol-lowering drug is usually considered as well. At the other end of the scale, adults with cholesterols above 200 mg-percent (and children with levels above 170 mg-percent) should not eat much animal fat (i.e: eggs, whole milk, butter, cream, cheese, meat fat, etc.) since their levels are likely to rise above 230, too, if they are not careful.

Fish Oil and Cholesterol

University of Oregon researchers have shown that fish oil

is better than vegetable oil at reducing high levels of lipid (fat and cholesterol) in the blood. Given as a supplement to people with hyperlipidemia (high blood lipids), the quantity of oil used was equivalent to eating about a pound of fish every day. This research, according to *Medical World News* (23#2:97), was prompted by the observation that Eskimos, who live largely on fish, almost never suffer from coronary heart disease.

Salmon oil (that can be taken as Maxepa capsules) is now widely accepted as a dietary means of both lowering the cholesterol blood level and preventing hardening of the arteries, thereby lowering the risks of heart attack and stroke. Each Maxepa capsule, according to the *Medical Letter* (24:99), contains 180 mg of the unsaturated fatty acid known as EPA (eicosapentaenoic acid), which is about one-tenth of the amount taken daily by people in research that demonstrated a beneficial effect. It remains to be seen, though, whether this much Maxepa (10 capsules a day, or a total of 1,800 mg daily), taken indefinitely, will prove to be safe. Since this substance is technically a "food," it has escaped the usual safety testing that the FDA requires for all new drugs.

In addition, it has been found, the active chemicals in salmon oil also slightly reduce the blood's ability to clot, correspondence in the *New England Journal of Medicine* (315:892) reports. However, with usual doses, this effect is not enough, by itself, to produce dangerous bleeding. Actually, the prolongation of the "bleeding time" test (following a finger prick) that occurs after large doses are taken daily for a month is smaller than occurs in response to treatment with one aspirin tablet.

Nevertheless, this cannot be ignored since, should both aspirin and salmon oil be taken together, their combined prolonging effect on bleeding might under certain circumstances be dangerous. Furthermore, as with aspirin, it would be wise to stop taking salmon oil two days or more prior to surgery.

The next article points out facts about other fish oil products.

Fish Oil Products Vary

Not all Omega-3 fish oil products are the same, even though the amounts of their cholesterol-lowering components (EPA and DCA) do not vary. Like old-fashioned cod liver oil, these products also contain some vitamin A and vitamin D, and in many cases some vitamin E as well.

If a product's label states that it contains 2 percent of the RDA (recommended daily allowance) for vitamins A and D, this is acceptable just so long as one is not already obtaining large doses of these vitamins from other sources.

However, many of these products contain quite a lot of vitamin E — as much as 6 percent of the RDA per capsule. This is a cause for concern. By taking 10 capsules of fish oil daily, one would get 60 percent of the RDA for vitamin E. That much vitamin E, added to the amount one gets from other sources, could easily be excessive and give rise to internal hemorrhaging. As we stated above, EPA (eicosapentaenoic acid), the major cholesterol-lowering ingredient of fish oil, already has a blood-thinning effect that could make internal bleeding in response to trauma more likely. By adding vitamin E's effect to this, we increase the risk of bleeding.

Some fish oil products, such as Maxepa, Proto-Chol and Promega, however, are free of vitamin E and seem to be more refined; their higher price can therefore be justified.

To be on the safe side, furthermore, it is advisable to limit one's intake of fish oil capsules to no more than 10 a day. This much EPA, *Drug Therapy* (17#2:53) reports, does not prolong the bleeding time (a test that measures the likelihood of internal hemorrhage). However, twice that number of fish oil capsules (20) every day does prolong the bleeding time beyond normal. We should take this matter very seriously because the Eskimos, whose diet contains large amounts of EPA, are protected from the dangers of cholesterol (such as heart attack), but die most often from bleeding within the brain (cerebral hemorrhage). Be careful, therefore, to buy only those fish oil capsules that are free of vitamin E and take no more of them than 10 each day.

Fish Oil Harmful for Diabetics

Since Omega-3 fish oil supplements help us to rid our bodies of cholesterol, it was hoped that they would be especially good for diabetics, whose arteries are prone to become choked with thick deposits of cholesterol. Now, unfortunately, *Medical World News* (28#11:104) reports, the omega-3 fish oils have been found to decrease the amount of insulin the body is capable of producing in response to food. This results in higher blood sugar levels after meals.

In that diabetics already have difficulty in producing insulin, fish oil supplements could make matters worse. Possibly, by taking more insulin, this difficulty could be overcome. Meanwhile, however, until more is known about this effect, it is safer for diabetics not to take capsules of fish oil at all.

High Fiber Diet

Despite their number and variety, all high fiber products have one thing in common: they are plant cell remnants that cannot be digested, the *U.S. Pharmacist* (12#7:42) reports. Without providing calories, they take up space in the stomach and intestines and thereby help to satisfy hunger.

Some, like wheat bran, increase the bulk of the stools but are sometimes constipating. Others, like oat bran, also tend to make the stools softer and more easily passed. Oat bran has a very useful cholesterol-lowering effect as well. For many, a mixture of these brans may be ideal. Salad, vegetables, and fruit (especially if unpeeled) also provide some dietary fiber.

Dietary fiber tends to bind onto other substances in the intestine and thereby prevents them (at least, in part) from being absorbed. This is one of the ways in which they help us to lose weight. However, fiber can also interfere with the absorption of some medications and essential nutrients (i.e., calcium). Accordingly, people who depend upon medicines for blood pressure, heart failure, or epilepsy, etc., or who are taking calcium for their bones should consult their doctors before starting a high fiber diet.

Pritikin Diet

Dr. Nathan Pritikin founded an institution named after him that champions both a diet that is high in fiber and low in fat and cholesterol, and a lifestyle that includes a lot of exercise. He died in 1985 from cancer. At autopsy, his heart and coronary arteries showed no trace of atherosclerosis ("hardening" from fat and cholesterol deposits), the *New England Journal of Medicine* (313:52) reports. This is remarkable because, 30 years earlier, before he started dieting and exercising, he had severe coronary disease, with dangerously high blood levels of cholesterol. By practicing what he preached, Dr. Pritikin rid himself completely of arterial disease and set a good example for us all.

Oats and Cholesterol

The trouble with most cholesterol-lowering diets, comments *Postgraduate Medicine* (77#8:29) is that they involve far too many *don'ts* and only a few *do's*.

Most of us find it difficult to reduce our intake of animal fats by significant amounts. Another problem we have is that, by increasing our intake of roughage (dietary fiber), we can only lower the blood cholesterol by about 10 percent. When the blood cholesterol level is dangerously high, of course, one has to take a cholesterol-lowering drug, and a few unlucky people need to do so all the time. But what should the average person wishing to lower the blood cholesterol do without resorting to medication?

The answer may well be that we should eat some whole oat bran regularly every day. According to the *American Journal of Clinical Nutrition* (40:1146), if we take about three and a half ounces of oat bran every day in the form of cereal and/or muffins (items sold in most supermarkets), most of us can easily bring the blood cholesterol level down by about 20 percent. This regimen should not be difficult to follow and is likely to be yet more effective if animal fats are also restricted, thereby in many cases making medicines for lowering cholesterol unnecessary. Cholesterol-lowering drugs, incidentally, tend to be expensive and to cause side effects.

Oat bran contains a vegetable fiber that is water soluble

and brings down cholesterol blood levels in several ways. First, it stimulates the liver to include more acid (produced by tearing down cholesterol) in the bowel juice that it secretes into the intestines. Second, oat fiber is broken down in the intestine into chemical fragments that, after being absorbed, inhibit cholesterol production by the tissues (cholesterol comes not only from our food but is also made by our own tissues).

According to *Postgraduate Medicine* (84#2:280), a carefully controlled study at the University of California compared the effects of oat bran with those of wheat bran, whole wheat flour, and a mixture of wheat and oat brans. Only oat bran brought about a significant drop in cholesterol and triglycerides. Interestingly, the amount of oat bran used in the study was only two rounded tablespoonfuls every day. No side effects were reported.

One wonders, though, whether some side effects would have been encountered if a larger amount of oat bran had been taken. Some people, as many as 15 percent in one survey, state that they are unable to take oat bran because it causes so much bloating and diarrhea. Possibly these people have been taking too much bran. They might well experience no bloating and diarrhea and derive just as much benefit, so far as cholesterol is concerned, if they were to take merely two rounded tablespoonfuls a day. Most good things are spoiled if taken in excess.

Oat bran reduces blood levels of cholesterol even in diabetics, who otherwise have trouble in keeping their cholesterol down at reasonable levels and are unusually prone to have cholesterol deposits in their arteries, with complications such as heart attack and stroke.

An oat bran hot cereal product is marketed by the Quaker Oats Company and is now available in many groceries and health food stores. With oat bran and salmon oil, we have two safe and very effective non-drug natural foodstuffs that can be used to control cholesterol.

Vitamin C Lowers Blood Cholesterol

Despite dieting, some people find it impossible to keep their blood cholesterol down to normal without medication. As we mentioned above, drugs used for this purpose are expensive, can be obtained only with a prescription, and sometimes cause serious side effects.

Now, according to correspondence in *Lancet*, vitamin C slowly but surely lowers the blood cholesterol without danger. In the past, not everyone agreed that vitamin C could do this, but recent studies with large numbers of patients of all kinds explain the diversity of opinion.

When the blood cholesterol is already within the normal range, vitamin C cannot force it any lower but, when it is above the normal range, vitamin C slowly reduces it toward normal. According to the report, one gram daily of vitamin C seems adequate. Once started, treatment for high blood cholesterol should be kept up for life.

Breakfast Cereals

Ready-to-eat breakfast cereals are tasty and convenient, but a lot of them are far from "healthy," according to *Consumer Reports* (CR) (51#10:628). Although their basic ingredients, such as corn, wheat, oats, raisins, and nuts are nutritious, many breakfast cereals contain excessive and potentially harmful amounts of saturated fat (i.e., in the form of coconut oil) and salt, which the manufacturers have added to make them more tasty and appealing.

Now, CR reports that the popular Quaker 100% Natural Cereal, because of its coconut content, provides an astonishing amount of saturated fat (the sort than can be responsible for high blood cholesterol levels, heart attacks, and strokes). The CR article also points out that most fiber and bran-containing ready-to-eat cereals provide salt or sugar (or both) in large amounts.

Fiber and bran products have become very popular since they have been shown to help fight constipation and cholesterol and to reduce the chance of our getting colon cancer. It is a pity, therefore, that these products should contain added salt, sugar, or fat in such large amounts.

With very little effort, however, we can prepare a high fiber cereal for ourselves that contains the most desirable water-soluble kind fiber, but no additives. Just boil water and stir in some powdered oat bran. This hot cereal will be free of sugar, salt, and fat, unless you add them to it yourself.

Coffee and Cholesterol

Reports about coffee and its effects upon the level of cholesterol in the blood have been alarmingly contradictory. Some researchers find that coffee, even in moderate amounts, raises cholesterol blood levels and thereby increases the risk of both heart attack and stroke. Others are unable to see any of these effects. Now, according to the *Lancet* (2:1283), there may be an explanation for these conflicting results.

The conflict began with a study by researchers in Norway in which they found that coffee drinking raised the blood levels of both cholesterol and fat. Furthermore, they discovered, the effect grew stronger the more cups of coffee the subjects consumed. In light of that, the *New England Journal of Medicine* (308:1454) said that heavy coffee drinkers probably at least incur double the risk of coronary artery disease. However, researchers in this country were unable to confirm these conclusions.

A new report says that the difference may lie in the variations in the methods by which the coffee was prepared for drinking. If coffee is made by boiling (as it was in the Norwegian study), there is a cholesterol-raising effect. In contrast, when our coffee is prepared by filtration (as it usually is nowadays in the U.S.A.), no bad effect on the blood cholesterol or the cardiovascular system is to be seen. Possibly, however, when we percolate coffee, although this is not proven, we may be producing at least some of the same undesirable effects as we would do if we boiled it.

Cream Substitutes

Those who limit their animal fat intake by substituting vegetable products for milk and cream may be interested to learn that many nondairy products of this sort contain coconut oil, palm oil, and palm kernel oil, all of which are rich in saturated fat.

Most vegetable and fish oils are unsaturated fats, the kind that is beneficial and that (unlike saturated animal fat) does not clog up the heart and arteries with atherosclerosis. However, coconut and palm oils, although of vegetable origin, are exceptions to the rule and are highly saturated fats of the kind normally found only in animal tissues, *Modern Medicine* (54#3:21) reports.

Use of nondairy creamers containing coconut or palm oils, therefore, is counterproductive if you are trying to avoid the danger of saturated fat. To avoid these oils, read the list of ingredients on all of the products you use.

Nicotine Acid Excess

While there is no doubt that dietary supplements of nicotinic acid help to lower the blood level of cholesterol, some people have been taking it in such excessively large doses that they have injured their livers.

The *Southern Medical Journal* (76:239) reports the case of a man who took about four grams (4,000 mg) of nicotinic acid daily for several months and became ill with fever, jaundice (yellowness of the skin), nausea, vomiting, and pain, swelling, and tenderness in the abdomen. Tests showed that his liver function was seriously disturbed. All of these problems quickly subsided after he stopped taking nicotinic acid.

However, not believing that a vitamin (nicotinic acid is a member of the vitamin B complex) could cause illness, he started taking large doses of nicotinic acid again a year later. Once more he suffered with the same symptoms, which were again proved to be due to liver toxicity, and which, for the second time, subsided when he stopped taking nicotinic acid.

The medical literature contains 11 more case reports of patients with liver disease who had been taking three to four grams of nicotinic acid daily. These doses are 30 to 40 times greater than the 100 mg daily doses recommended as an adjunct in controlling the blood cholesterol. Limiting one's intake of animal fat and cholesterol, however, must remain the cornerstone of any program to prevent atherosclerosis.

Chromium

By supplementing our diets with chromium, according to the *Journal of the American Medical Association* (247:3046), we may improve the manner in which our bodies handle sugar. Whether obtained from brewer's yeast or from tablets of inorganic chromium, the supplement works by optimizing the production and effects of insulin, with which "normal" (non-diabetic) people dispose of sugar.

In addition, researchers have shown, chromium helps to normalize the serum cholesterol, increasing its "good" HDL fraction while reducing the "bad" LDL. Chromium is naturally present in wine and also in some brands of beer. Perhaps this is the mechanism, the *Journal* speculates, whereby a little wine every day helps to reduce the incidence of fatal heart attack.

COLON PROBLEMS

Testing for Colon Cancer

As we have reported before, a huge number of unnecessary deaths from colon cancer could be prevented if people routinely had their stools tested for blood for three days every year.

One can easily perform the test by oneself at home with a kit that is mailed to a laboratory. The kits, instructions for use, and mailers can be obtained from most doctors. If any of the three tests turn out to be positive, the person is advised to avoid red meat, raw vegetables, and iron-containing medicines for another three days, after which the testing is repeated. If any of the second series of tests is positive, the person is advised to visit a doctor for further investigation, such as X-rays and inspection of the colon through an instrument.

By these means about 95 percent of colorectal cancers can be detected early enough to be cured. The latest news on this appeared in the *New England Journal of Medicine* (312:1448), which mentioned another precaution that needs to be taken. To avoid "false negative" results, vitamin C supplements should not be taken for a few days before and during the time when one is testing the stools for blood. In other words, taking vitamin C during the tests can make it appear that one's stools are free of blood when, in fact, they are not, so that a diagnosis of cancer can be missed.

Diverticulosis

Whereas only one in 10 Americans has developed diverticulosis by the age of 40, about two out of three does so by age 60. Most people with this condition, fortunately, never know that there is anything wrong, *Drug Therapy* (17#6:53) reports.

That is not surprising since diverticulosis is nothing more than a series of little pouches hanging from the wall of the colon. These are really just hernias from the lining of the colon which become pushed out after the colon has repeatedly strained to propel hard stools.

If symptoms do occur, they include tenderness of the left lower abdomen, cramping, bloating, nausea, vomiting, and constipation (sometimes alternating with diarrhea). Problems arise when the content of the intestine cannot easily be moved along the colon, and some of it is forced into the pouches, which then become plugged and infected.

Once diverticulosis has developed, nothing can be done to reverse it. Nevertheless, plenty of fluid and enough of the right foods (e.g., oat bran, whole meal bread, fruit, and vegetables) in one's diet will usually prevent constipation. A dietitian could give helpful advice. Exercise, too, for reasons that are not well understood, is definitely helpful. Lastly, laxatives and enemas, because they irritate the colon, tend to do more harm than good for people with diverticulosis.

Constipation

Many factors may contribute to constipation, the *American Family Physician* (27#1:179) suggests, including lack of exercise, decreased appetite and thirst, and too great a reliance upon commercially prepared low bulk foods. When not disease-related, constipation should respond readily to taking extra fluid and bulk with every meal and, if necessary, a stool softener medication such as Colace, Doxidan, or Surfak.

These drugs are not effective alone and must always be taken with bran, or a lubricant (such as mineral oil), or both. When bran is added to the diet, calcium, phosphorus, and iron are trapped in the gut by the undigested cellulose. This could be a factor in the bone thinning in some of the elderly, who already have difficulty in maintaining a positive calcium balance. Calcium and iron supplements are therefore essential if one is taking bran. Also, since mineral oil traps fat-soluble vitamins, one should try to compensate for this by taking mineral oil and vitamins at different times of day.

DEAFNESS AND EAR PROBLEMS

Noise-induced Deafness

Hardness of hearing in older persons most often results from their having been repeatedly exposed, over a lifetime, to very loud noise. Inner ear damage produced by "acoustic trauma," unfortunately, is permanent and cumulative, and the hearing loss it causes develops progressively over a period of decades.

Although Americans are now protected by law from excessive noise in the workplace, many of us nevertheless continue to damage our hearing permanently by noisy leisure activities, *Emergency Medicine* (20#11:169) reports. Firing guns, listening to loud rock music, or operating unmuffled lawn mowers, motorcycles, snowmobiles, etc., are typical of the means by which people slowly but surely lose much of their hearing. While a single shotgun blast close to the ear can cause lasting deafness, the effects of most other types of loud noise are not so immediately apparent, and people continue to expose themselves to it again and again.

For this reason, *Geriatrics* (37#8:107) recommends, we should always wear ear mufflers to protect our hearing every time we mow the lawn, use a chain saw, shoot, or drive a noisy vehicle, etc. In older persons, this is more important than ever, especially when there is already some hearing loss. Even the young, when exposed to loud noise (this includes music), are unlikely to escape this effect.

Merely putting cotton or paper in the ears while performing noisy tasks does no good because one needs plugs that fit the canals snugly. Large muffs that completely cover the ears can be counted upon for protection and are much more convenient.

Certain medicines and alcohol magnify the risk of hearing loss from noise.

Zinc and Hearing

Older patients with tinnitus (ringing ears) and hearing loss due to degeneration of the inner ear, in many cases, have fully recovered following treatment with zinc sulfate, 600 mg daily. A doctor at Northwestern University Medical School, according to a report in *Geriatrics* (38#4:21), has brought about complete remission of these inner ear disease symptoms in 20 patients so far with zinc. Other signs of zinc deficiency mentioned in the report include hair loss, diminished sense of taste and smell, fragile nails, rough skin, adult acne, and slow wound healing. Because they can be harmful to the liver, doses of zinc larger than 220 mg daily should not be taken for longer than necessary.

Middle Ear Infections and Hearing Loss

In a Harvard study, according to *Modern Medicine*, it was found that 10 percent of children are partially deaf for three months after middle ear infections, and those who have repeated infections may be hard of hearing for seven to eight months every year. Children who recover from earache and fever usually do not complain if they have some lingering deafness, even when it is bad enough to create problems at school. The common assumption is that they are not concentrating or are not smart enough to keep up. Adults, particularly older ones, can have this problem, too.

Beta-Blocker Deafness

Beta-blockers, such as propranolol and metoprolol, are very popular medications for high blood pressure and a number of diseases of the heart. Their side effects, including weakness, slow pulse, an unpleasant sensation in the chest during exercise when the heart is not quite able to pump fast enough to meet the body's increased demands, and even an occasional case of arthritis, have been well-documented.

Deafness, however, has only rarely been described, and a report in the *British Medical Journal* (289:1490) adds another case to the series. It is an important case because it suggests that treatment with a beta-blocker may often be overlooked as the cause of deafness, which has all the symptoms of a problem in the middle ear (just inside the eardrum).

Possibly, these drugs cause arthritis of the joints between the middle ear ossicles, the three tiny bones that magnify sound-induced vibrations of the eardrum and convey them to the inner ear's organ of hearing. This idea is not so far-fetched since beta-blockers do sometimes cause arthritis between the bones of other joints. Furthermore, like arthritis that is caused by beta-blockers, the deafness described in the *Journal* cleared up in a few weeks after the drug had been discontinued.

The moral of this story, therefore, is to stop taking a beta-blocker (if possible) just as soon as deafness appears since, if the drug is contained, more permanent hearing loss may occur. Fortunately, other drugs can be used in most cases. Since diseases for which beta-blockers are needed are often serious, the doctor who ordered the drug must be consulted before any change is made.

Deafness with Flying

Earache and deafness occur whenever the air pressure in the middle ear differs from that of our surroundings. One of the most common causes of this is the rapid change in altitude when we are flying. We obtain relief by swallowing, yawning, or by "popping the ears." These help by momentarily opening the eustachian canals (passageways connecting the back of the throat with the middle ears), allowing air to move into or out of the ears to equalize the pressure on either side of the eardrums. Two things can interfere with popping the ears, *Emergency Medicine* (14#8:155) points out: swelling of the mucous membranes with a cold or allergy, and being too young to do it properly. Small children, who might otherwise suffer while flying, can help themselves by blowing up a balloon or two, especially during landings.

DEPRESSION

Depression and Other Diseases

Depression is a physical disease that, among other things, causes the victim to be sad and withdrawn. Because it often not only affects the mind but also interferes with the function of other parts of the body as well, physicians refer to it as the "great imitator". Thus, many older people who are thought to have Alzheimer's disease (senile dementia) may, instead, actually be depressed. This is so in about 25 percent of "dementia" cases, *Geriatrics* (42#4:53) reports.

The big difference between these conditions is that depression begins suddenly whereas Alzheimer's dementia comes on gradually over a period of years. Even though both disorders tend to affect behavior in the same way, it is important to distinguish between them since depression often responds to medication, whereas Alzheimer's disease is irreversible.

Depression, too, often occurs as a complication of disabling illness, such as a heart attack or stroke, when it tends to interfere with recovery. For example, according to the *Lancet* (1:743), stroke victims with depression generally remain severely impaired after two years, whereas equally severe stroke patients who are not depressed are much more likely to regain use of their limbs and the power of speech. However, unless one thinks of the possibility, depression in stroke victims can easily be overlooked.

Exercise Treatment for Depression

Exercising regularly and intensely enough to increase the pulse rate and make oneself short of breath, many physicians believe, will help a person overcome mental depression. Although there is no scientific proof for this, the *Physician and Sportsmedicine* (13#9:192) reports, many psychologists and psychiatrists are sufficiently convinced of a beneficial relationship between hard exercise and a positive frame of mind that they now recommend it routinely for all of their depressed patients if there is no health contraindication.

Mental depression of the type that responds to exercise (reactive depression) is defined as a feeling of sadness greater and more prolonged than is warranted by its cause. It is characterized by sadness, dullness, immobility, a sense of helplessness, and loss of self esteem. Depression that occurs without a triggering event and as a part of a severe mental illness (psychosis) will never respond to exercise alone, but requires psychotherapy and special medication.

One need not be a jogger or runner to overcome reactive depression, it has been found, and people who regularly engage in such activities as tennis, walking long distances, swimming, or rowing can benefit. To be of value, however, the exercise should be a kind that is somewhat demanding and also improves physical fitness

DIABETES

Diabetes and Sugar

Until recently, much importance was attached to restricting the use of sugar in the treatment of diabetes. Today, therefore, it is surprising to hear certain experts say that sugars, like sucrose and fructose, can safely be added as sweeteners to the food of diabetics. This is still controversial.

An article in *British Medical Journal* (288:1025) suggests that it is premature to recommend sugar for diabetics simply on the basis of short-term blood level studies after test meals sweetened with sucrose or fructose. Rather, the *Journal* recommends, we should wait and see what happens when sugars have been added to the diets of a limited number of diabetic volunteers for several years. Possibly, the long-term effect may not be desirable.

Meanwhile, it is recommended that diabetics avoid simple sugars. Complex carbohydrates, however, especially the bulk-providing ones such as beans, peas, bran, wholemeal bread, and natural cereals are acceptable in that they do not quickly release a lot of sugar during digestion. In fact, they even reduce the need for insulin by trapping sugar in the gut. Furthermore, by providing calories that might otherwise have to be supplied by fat and meat (which provide cholesterol), complex carbohydrates can help to prevent atherosclerosis, the major complication of diabetes.

Diabetes and Alcohol

An important news item for diabetics in the *British Medical Journal* (288:1035) is the discovery that alcohol usage helps to bring on proliferative retinitis, the most common cause of blindness in diabetics. The retina is the light-detecting nerve layer in the back of the eye. Alcohol usage was defined as taking at least 10 drinks (beers, glasses of wine, shots of whiskey, gin, etc.) per week. Since alcohol is a close relative of glucose, one could imagine that it is bad for diabetics in two ways — both as a sugar and as a toxic agent for nerve cells, including those in the eye.

DIARRHEA

Severe Diarrhea Caused by Sweetener

Because of the saccharin ban, food manufacturers are now

using sorbitol as a low-calorie sugar substitute. Although chemically related to sugar, sorbitol is neither broken down nor absorbed by the human body. Furthermore, like saccharin, it does not promote tooth decay, and is therefore also used as a sweetener in chewing gum, breath mints, and certain candies.

Now — a word of warning. According to a letter in the *Journal of the American Medical Association,* sorbitol can produce severe side effects. During a two hour medical meeting, a physician ate one roll of 12 sorbitol-containing, mint flavored candies. Half an hour later, he experienced swelling and cramping pain in the abdomen, with the passage of excessive gas rectally. During the next few hours, he developed such severe diarrhea that he collapsed and was admitted to hospital. The abdominal pain became so severe that a perforated gastric ulcer was suspected. Fortunately, this proved not to be so, and he recovered in 24 hours.

Because it is not absorbed from the stomach or intestines, sorbitol, in large doses, acts like Epsom salts and pulls water into the intestines from the blood stream. This, in turn, prevents absorption of food, which ferments and produces excessive gas, bloating, and diarrhea. Adults, and especially small children, beware! Read the list of ingredients on candy and gum wrappers. If the product contains sorbitol, take no more than one piece an hour and try to make a roll of 12 pieces last all day.

Dysentery from Hamburger Meat

Although the first several victims reported in a recent dysentery outbreak had all eaten hamburgers in two restaurants of the same fast food chain, it soon became evident that similar cases were occurring all over the country and involved people who had eaten hamburger meat at home. Typical cases, according to *Internal Medicine Alert* (4:79), experienced abdominal cramps, severe enough to be compared with childbirth, and bloody diarrhea. There was no fever. The cause was discovered to be bacteria that can survive partial cooking and which grow particularly well in ground beef. Protect yourself by eating only hamburgers that are well done.

Sickroom Fluids May Be Hazardous

Drinking to replace fluid lost by diarrhea, vomiting, or sweating seems nothing more than common sense. Even so, there is danger in this simple treatment. The problem, according to *Emergency Medicine*, arises when the fluid contains too much sugar or too much salt. If the fluid is too strong, it is not absorbed and dilutes itself by attracting liquid out of the patient's tissues until it reaches equilibrium with the salt or sugar content of the patient's blood. Strong fluids, even fruit juice or canned soup, can actually worsen dehydration. So, when the doctor orders fruit juices or clear fluids for someone sick at home, reconstitute them with twice as much water as the label recommends, and avoid salty soups entirely.

Cholera Mystery Solved

Cholera is a dreaded epidemic disease that causes such violent diarrhea that its victims may die from dehydration a few hours after they begin to feel unwell. Occurring mostly in tropical countries which have poor hygiene, cholera classically spreads from person to person in contaminated drinking water.

In the last few years, however, small cholera outbreaks have occurred in Europe in places where the hygiene is above reproach. Until recently, these little epidemics could not be explained, but now we may have the answer.

Liquid effluents from passenger planes, it has been found, produce small droplets of water in the air that gradually drift down to the earth. Although most aircraft have chemical holding tanks for semi-solid sewage, nearly all planes discharge water directly into the air from lavatory basins and spill liquid overflow from their tanks.

Experiments reported in the *Journal of Hygiene*, furthermore, indicate that even the water drops released by planes flying high in the stratosphere can carry live bacteria and viruses down to the ground, thereby posing a health hazard. Incidentally, the European communities affected by cholera lie directly under the flight path of jets traveling from India, where cholera is a common cause of death.

Another mystery was recently solved in South Africa, where gold miners unaccountably came down with cholera despite high standards of purity in their drinking water and food. There, according to *The New Scientist*, bacteria-containing water droplets got into the mine's air supply from a cholera-carrying visitor's sweat and were disseminated by ventilator fans.

Since dangerous germs spread with such frightening ease almost anywhere in the world, avoid touching food and putting your fingers in your mouth without first washing your hands, wherever you are.

DIZZINESS

Causes of Dizziness

Apart from the unpleasantness and inconvenience, dizzy spells catch people off guard and can result in fractures. The causes of dizziness, according to *Geriatrics* (37#4:117), may involve almost any part of the body, including especially the ear, nerves, brain, heart, and circulatory system. Some are difficult to detect because they occur only during dizzy spells and at other times leave no trace.

For example, one of the most common causes of dizziness is an abnormal heart rhythm that lasts for just a few seconds. During that time, the heart pumps so inefficiently that it fails to deliver an adequate blood supply to the brain. To detect such transient and occasional arrhythmias, the patient may need to wear a Holter Monitor (a tiny, portable electrocardiograph machine) for days on end while going about life normally at home. Most such heart rhythm disturbances, when detected and studied, can be controlled with medication.

Other causes of dizzy spells range from the very simple (hard wax, a hair, or some other "foreign body" touching the ear drum) to the rather complex (the low blood sugar that can occur following meals in "pre-diabetes").

Dizziness that keeps occurring without apparent cause often makes people fearful and depressed, and one must not give up too quickly in searching for the cause.

DRUG AND MEDICINE PROBLEMS

Drug Side Effects in the Elderly

Adverse reactions to medications are much more likely to occur and to be serious in older people than in the young, the *American Family Physician* (34#6:118) reports. In several studies of elderly people, an adverse reaction was found to be the cause of admission to the hospital in 25 to 40 percent of cases.

The reasons for this common problem are various, and one cannot single out anything that applies to them all. Nevertheless, many drugs can cause nutritional depletion by interfering with the absorption of food and the sense of taste. This, in turn can lead to a deficiency of vitamin C, which makes such people much more prone to stomach injury by aspirin and anti-arthritis drugs, with gastric ulcer and internal bleeding as the result.

Blood pressure medicines, water pills (diuretics), and pain drugs can all produce lightheadedness and fainting when one stands up, leading to falls and injuries. Blood pressure medicines are also a very common cause of mental depression. Because side effects so often simulate natural illness, anyone who begins to feel unwell while taking medication should wonder whether the drug is to blame and should ask the pharmacist or doctor what to do.

Some medicines, such as cimetidine (trade-named Tagamet), can impair the liver's ability to chemically dispose of other drugs. This is because the liver steadily decreases in 40 percent smaller than that of a young adult. On top of this, by virtue of hardening of the arteries, the liver's blood supply tends to be reduced, thereby further impairing the organ's ability to break down and dispose of drugs.

While aging, there is also a reduction in the amount of blood circulating through the kidneys. Since many drugs are eliminated from the body in proportion to the kidney's blood flow, here is another good reason for the elderly to take reduced doses.

A recent editorial in *Geriatrics* (38#11:39) concluded that elderly persons often cannot tolerate the "usual adult dosage" that is recommended on the labels of most medicine bottles. In view of what we now know, this is understandable. When in doubt, therefore, it is usually safer for older persons to take only about half the usual adult dose. However, if a drug is prescribed by the doctor, take it as ordered, but then ask him to confirm that the dosage is appropriate for your age, if you are over 65.

Joint Problems and Heart Medication

An article in *British Medical Journal* (287:1256) reports the case of a man who developed pain and swelling in both knees while taking the beta blocker drug practolol to prevent a recurrence of heart attack. His symptoms subsided when he stopped the drug but promptly recurred when he started it again.

Looking for similar cases, his doctor found 18 others whose joints were affected by beta blockers, which they were taking for blood pressure or heart disease. Many were on propranolol, another beta blocker.

The most commonly affected joints were the shoulders (13 patients), and the knees (six). Five had generalized joint problems and two had pain and swelling of their fingers, like those of rheumatoid arthritis. Nevertheless, this was much milder than rheumatoid arthritis or osteoarthritis and always cleared up, quickly and completely, when the beta blocker drug was discontinued.

The doctor reporting this experience believes it may be a common side effect that is usually assumed to be natural arthritis. He suspects that it may be due to a drying effect of beta blockers in the joints, which are naturally lubricated with a slippery fluid. Beta blockers, incidentally, have a drying effect on other moist surfaces, such as those of the eye, nose, and mouth. So, if you develop joint pains while taking a beta blocker, you need not be too concerned.

Commonly Used Antibiotic Sometimes Causes Brain Swelling

Tetracycline, the antibiotic taken by thousands of teen-agers for acne, is a rare but well-known cause of brain swelling in infants, making the soft, non-bony parts of their heads (the fontanelles) bulge outward. This side effect usually disap-pears within a day or two if the tetracycline is discontinued right away.

For about 25 years, tetracycline-associated brain swelling was regarded as a problem peculiar to infancy, but now, according to the *British Medical Journal* (262:19), it has also been discovered in adults. Since, unlike babies, adults have no soft parts in the skull, there is no tell-tale bulging of the head to help diagnose this condition after infancy. Adults, do, however, have headache, blurred vision, nausea, and vomit-ing.

Alarming, but not serious, this swelling subsides just as

promptly in adults as it does in babies after tetracycline is discontinued. To date, there has been no suggestion of tetra-cycline-associated brain damage, but, just to make sure, stop taking the drug, and consult your physician right away for an alternative antibiotic if you develop a headache while on tet-racycline.

Side Effects of Valium

According to research reported in the *British Medical Journal* (283:343), Valium (diazepam) may actually worsen the anxiety associated with shortness of breath due to emphy-sema (the permanent lung damage that may occur in smokers). Being a tranquilizer, Valium also relaxes muscles, an effect that robs emphysema victims of the strength they need in their continuous struggle for breath. Anything that relaxes muscles, and this includes sleeping pills and alcohol, should be avoided by those who are always short of breath.

Another side effect of Valium that has been encountered by men of all ages is breast enlargement of almost feminine proportions. In four out of five with this side effect, reported in the *Lancet* (2:1225), the breasts slowly decreased in size after Valium was discontinued. Not usually accompanied by impotence or any other gender-related problems, this breast enlargement was believed due to Valium-induced chemical changes in the tissues in which testosterone (male hormone) became converted into estradiol (a female hormone).

Since Valium is currently America's most widely pre-scribed medication, and we have not heard about this before, the incidence must be quite low. Nevertheless, men needing a tranquilizer might wish to try something other than Valium.

Alcohol and Acetaminophen

Acetaminophen, the non prescription pain-killer that has weathered the storm of two capsule tampering scares, is currently being talked about for a more basic reason, *Medical World News* (27#8:56) reports.

Liver specialists are concerned about the lack of guidelines on the safe upper limit of acetaminophen dosage that can be taken by those who drink alcohol regularly. Everyone agrees that those who drink quite a lot of alcohol every day are at a greater than normal risk of acetaminophen-induced inflammation of the liver, which sometimes results in death from liver failure. Alcohol induces acetaminophen to be broken down by the body in an unusual way, which results in production of chemicals that are poisonous to the liver.

Experts agree that, in the presence of alcoholism, even reasonably conventional doses of acetaminophen can be dangerous. They differ, however, on the amount of acetaminophen that can be safely taken by people who merely drink some alcohol every day, but who are by no means "alcoholics."

The most conservative opinion stated on this so far is that people who regularly drink at least three or four beers every day should never take more than two grams of acetaminophen during any 24-hour period. A glass of wine or of any other alcoholic drink would be the equivalent of one beer.

Enteric-Coated Aspirin

Aspirin is generally acknowledged to be an excellent pain reliever and, in large enough doses, performs no less well than the newer nonsteroidal anti-inflammatory drugs (NSAIDs), such as Clinoril, Motrin, Naprosyn, Nalfon, Rufen, Tolectin, etc., in relieving the pain, stiffness, and swelling of arthritic joints. The trouble is that, in high doses, aspirin can also be highly irritating to the stomach, even causing gastric ulcers with heavy bleeding. For this reason, more than anything else, doctors prefer to use the other drugs (listed above), which are thought to be less irritating to the stomach.

To get around the gastric irritation problem, many arthritis specialists have started using enteric coated tablets of aspirin, which cannot dissolve in the acid of the stomach. These tablets do not begin disintegrating until they pass through the stomach and reach the intestines, where the juices are alkaline, and where the coating quickly dissolves and releases the aspirin.

Given as treatment to a group of elderly arthritis patients in Georgia, the *Southern Medical Journal* (76#2:276) reports, enteric coated aspirin proved to be a good substitute for NSAID tablets in 40 out of 42 cases and did not cause gastric problems in any of them. Aspirin is much less likely to injure the kidneys, liver, or bone marrow than are any of the NSAID drugs and, even when enteric coated, is very much less expensive ($3.50-$7.50 per month, as compared to $20-$45 per month for NSAIDs).

Aspirin — the Cause of Reye Syndrome?

Reye Syndrome, an uncommon complication of viral illnesses, most often of influenza or chickenpox, usually affects children aged between 5 and 11, and sometimes also young adults.

Presenting with severe vomiting, followed by lethargy, changes in personality, and then coma and even death, Reye Syndrome is due to inflammation, with swelling and disordered function of the brain and the liver. The cause of this complication has remained a mystery until now. The Public Health Service's *Morbidity and Mortality Weekly Report* (27:532) cites two studies, in Ohio and Michigan, both of which point to aspirin as a likely major factor. Aspirin's use in febrile illnesses, according to the report, increases the likelihood of Reye Syndrome about 11-fold.

If this is true, what should we do about the fever and discomfort of viral illnesses? Perhaps we should do nothing, suggests *Internal Medicine Alert* (2:71). Reducing fever may be counter-productive, *IMA* reports, since fever is one of nature's best defenses against the multiplication and spread of viruses in the body. Aspirin, therefore, while making febrile patients feel better, may actually prolong their illnesses and increase the likelihood of complications.

Please note, this does not apply to the small daily aspirin doses thought to be useful in reducing the likelihood of strokes and heart attacks.

Oral Polio Vaccine

Since it is made with modified but still "live" virus, oral polio vaccine (OPV) sometimes actually causes paralytic polio, the very illness it is supposed to prevent. Injectable polio vaccine (IPV), which is made with killed virus, cannot do this. In *Morbidity and Mortality Weekly Report* (31:22), the U.S. Public Health Service warns that OPV occasionally endangers not only those who are vaccinated with it but also, for a month afterwards, certain persons living in close contact with them. Anyone with deficient immunity is at risk, and this involves, among others, all cancer or leukemia patients, persons treated with radiation, or anyone taking cortisone-like steroid drugs, whether for arthritis, asthma, or any other ailment.

Since, even though rare, polio paralysis can cripple or kill, the Swedish government has now banned OPV. For the same reason, many American physicians prefer IPV, but, surprisingly, OPV continues to be the most widely used vaccine for polio in the U.S.A.

Help the Medicine Go Down

At the best of times, even when we are up and about, some of us have difficulty in swallowing tablets or capsules and getting them to go all the way down into the stomach. Medicines that get held up in the esophagus (the tubular structure that conveys food and drink from the throat down into the stomach) may not only delay the effectiveness of the medicine, but also may cause inflammation and ulceration of the esophagus. This is a condition that is medically known as esophagitis, and causes chest pain and vomiting.

Difficulty in swallowing pills is more likely to occur when one is in bed. Taking medicine when lying down, or lying down immediately after taking it, the *British Medical Journal* (285:1702) reports, results in pills or capsules "sticking" in the esophagus. To overcome the problem, a letter to the editor of the *Journal of the American Medical Association* (264:3425) suggests that, after we swallow pills that could stick in the esophagus, we should take some banana and chew it well. The pulpy fruit sweeps the esophagus clean as it descends. In addition, tablets or capsules should always be swallowed with half a glassful of water, and the pill-taker should stand or sit up for at least a quarter of a minute after taking medication.

EYESIGHT

Sunlight and Eye Problems

Malignant melanoma, a cancer that grows from pigment cells either of the skin or of the eye, is about three times more common in our southern states than in the North, the *New England Journal of Medicine* (313:789) reports, and the factor responsible seems to be the ultraviolet light in sunshine.

Not surprisingly, therefore, people with brown eyes (whose eyes are protected by the pigment) are only about half as likely as those who are blue-eyed to develop a melanoma of the eye. Furthermore, those who do develop this cancer are likely to have spent more time farming, gardening, or sunbathing outside, or tanning indoors with a lamp. Lastly, the report indicates the importance of protecting our eyes with a hat, visor, or sunglasses, which, if used routinely, reduce the risk of eye cancer by about 50 percent. Clearly, therefore, sunlight is a big factor in eye cancer, but one we can largely avoid. UV-filtering sunglasses should be worth their extra cost!

Sunlight is also an important factor in the development of cataracts, the *Western Journal of Medicine* (143:511) reports. Ultraviolet light (UV) causes the deposition of minute granules of an opaque brown pigment in the normally clear and colorless body of the lens. After many years, if the eyes continue to be exposed to strong sunshine, more and more granules are deposited until the lens becomes completely opaque, with blindness as a result. Vision can be instantly restored, of course, by surgically removing these cataracts and replacing them with artificial lenses.

The more we expose our eyes to UV, it has been found, the more opaque our lenses become. Not surprisingly, therefore, cataracts are much more common in the tropics than in the temperate zones of Europe and North America. Furthermore, they are less common in office workers than among people who work outside.

Along the same line, the *British Medical Journal* (65:869) reports that in the tropics people need reading glasses at an earlier age than they do in a cold climate. The average age at which glasses are first needed varies from 36 at one climatic extreme to 50 at the other. Again, stronger light could well be the factor involved, and people should be careful to wear sunglasses when exposed to bright sunlight.

A New Test for the Endangered Red Eye

When an eye is red as the result of trauma or infection, the danger of permanent visual damage is always greater if the inflammation has spread inwards far enough to involve the iris (the colored part of the eye). Detection of iritis (an inflamed iris) has traditionally required examination by an eye specialist.

Now, according to *Medical World News* (23#4:36), iritis can be diagnosed more easily. Just cover the affected eye with your hand, and then momentarily flash a light into the other eye. If pain occurs in the covered eye, this means that its iris is inflamed.

This simple test exploits the fact that the irises of both eyes move in unison in response to bright light, making both pupils smaller at the same time. If the iris is inflamed, pain occurs as the pupil constricts. Therefore, when you have a red eye and this light test proves "positive," make sure to get medical attention right away. Even if the test is negative, but you feel that all is not well, see your doctor anyway.

Cataract Prevention, Yet Another Use for Aspirin?

Physicians at Yale University Medical School have found a lower than expected incidence of cataract (visual difficulty due to cloudiness in the lens of the eye) among arthritis patients who had taken aspirin for many years. In arthritis patients who had not taken aspirin, cataract was as common as usual. This protective effect, according to *Internal Medicine Alert* (2:77), was even more pronounced in patients with diabetes, a condition which greatly increases the prevalence of cataracts, but cataracts were present in seven of eight diabetics whose arthritis had been managed without aspirin.

Aspirin, taken in the high doses used for arthritis, causes many more side effects than most physicians would care to accept in a treatment used only for prevention. Long-term studies in people without arthritis are therefore needed to determine whether small, better-tolerated doses of aspirin can also prevent cataract. Because this form of blindness is so common in the elderly, the project should get priority.

Vitamin C Probably Helps Prevent Cataracts

Researchers at the University of Maryland, according to the *Archives of Internal Medicine* (140:1269), have found that, in vitamin C deficiency, exposure to light of no greater intensity than that required for reading produces a damaging chemical in the lens of the eye. The photochemical end product, a superoxide, is closely akin to ozone, which can damage any living tissue.

Since the lens has no blood vessels (which would deprive it of transparency), locally made superoxides, unable to be carried away by the circulation, accumulate and have a more than usually damaging effect. Accumulation in the lens alters its chemical nature, making it less transparent, and thereby produces a cataract and blindness. The research strongly suggests that, by taking extra vitamin C, we can help prevent blindness due to cataracts. Cataracts have many causes, but this could be the most common one in people with poor nutrition.

Microwave Popcorn Danger to the Eyes

Steam released on opening food packages that have been heated by microwaves can be the cause of burns, correspondence in the *New England Journal of Medicine* (315:1359) points out. The letter reports a 10-year-old boy whose eyes and eyelids were damaged by the rush of steam released from a popcorn package that he was opening close to his face. The help of an eye specialist was required. Although the labels on such packages state: "Handle the bag carefully — It's hot," these words do not really warn the consumer about any danger to the eyes.

Senile Macular Degeneration, an Easy Test

If detected early enough, senile macular degeneration (SMD), the leading cause of blindness in the elderly, can be treated quite easily in the eye specialist's office with a laser beam. Treatment delayed for longer than two weeks after the first symptoms appear helps only about 10 percent of patients,

Geriatrics (37#12:21) reports, whereas treatment started earlier prevents progression of SMD in over 80 percent.

So important is early detection and treatment that it is a good idea for the elderly to check their vision daily for this potential problem. The test can be quickly performed without anybody's help or any special equipment. Merely stare, one eye at a time (covering the other with your hand), at a long straight line, such as a door frame. If, to either eye, the line appears bent or twisted, or if a black spot gets in the way, tell an ophthalmologist about it right away.

Night Shortsightedness

Many people who have perfect vision in daylight have difficulty in focusing clearly upon distant objects at night. Known as night myopia, this problem often begins with headaches and fear of driving after dark, the *American Family Physician* (31#6:105) reports.

The trouble is that vision is usually tested either in daylight or in strong artificial light, conditions under which night myopia cannot ordinarily be detected. Of course, if patients tell the eye doctor that they are having difficulty in seeing after dark, appropriate tests can then be made.

Night myopia must not be confused with night blindness, a temporary disorder of the retina that is due to deficiency of vitamin A. Night myopia is permanent and occurs in those who, even by day, are almost, but not quite, in need of spectacles for distant vision.

For mechanical reasons, when the lighting is poor, the lens has more difficulty than usual in changing its shape to focus upon objects at a distance. This is because the iris widens in the darkness to admit more light into the eye and thereby gets in the way of the moving lens. Night myopia is easily treated with spectacles that need be worn only when one is driving after dark.

Impotence From Eye Drops

Since they can be counted upon to reduce the ocular pressure, eyedrops that contain the beta-blocker drug timolol (trade name Timoptic in the U.S.A.) have become one of the most popular drugs for glaucoma, a letter to the editor of the *Journal of the American Medical Association* (253:3092) states. Not surprisingly, therefore, there have been many reports of side effects with timolol eyedrops, 63 percent of which have occurred after the drug has been absorbed into the general circulation. Among these, there have been cases of impotence, some of which have lasted (while the patient continued using the eyedrops) for over four years. Almost invariably, the impotence promptly disappears if the drops are discontinued, only to occur again when they are reinstated. The moral of this story is that anyone who becomes impotent should suspect that a medication could be responsible, even if eyedrops are the only one they are taking.

Administering Eye Drops

Many children, and even some adults, find it almost impossible to relax their lids when eye drops are being given. Even when they wish to cooperate, their lids are held so tightly shut that the drops fail to get into the eyes and drip down the cheeks instead. A good way to get around this problem, *Emergency Medicine* (16#14:170) suggests, is to ask the patient to lie down on his back and close his eyes. One or two drops of the medication are then put on the lids where they meet in a hollow at the nasal side of the eyes (the inner canthus), and the patient is then asked to blink. By gravity, and without any struggle, the drops will then run into the eyes as the lids are opened.

The Aging Eye

As we age, our eyes change in several ways that make vision less clear. Many of the changes are unavoidable, but, since excessive light exposure is known to accelerate cataract formation and to damage the retina (both of which occur with aging), we should at least try to slow these effects of aging as much as possible by regularly wearing proper sunglasses whenever we are outdoors.

Another thing that we can do to help ourselves is to have eye tests regularly for glaucoma, a condition that becomes more likely if we take certain medicines, including antihistamines, cough medicine, some types of sleeping pills, antidepressants, and drugs for dizziness or Parkinson's disease, *Postgraduate Medicine* (81#2:108) reports. These medications do not cause glaucoma but can aggravate it if it already exists. Furthermore, since these medicines are often essential, never discontinue them on this account without a doctor's orders. If you are taking one of these medicines, regular glaucoma testing is especially important.

Dry Eyes

As a "normal" effect of aging, almost everyone over 60 experiences some dryness of the eyes, *Geriatrics* (39#1:56) reports, and many are affected at an even younger age. Plenty of tears are still produced, but they lack their normal content of mucus and, consequently, no longer properly lubricate the cornea (the transparent front part of the eye).

Redness, itching, dryness, and a feeling as if there were grit in the eyes result. Worse yet, the front of the cornea becomes dried out in places, making vision slightly hazy from time to time. To overcome this, victims of sicca (the medical term for dry eye) frequently rub their eyes to spread tears over these dried out spots. In compensation, tears are then produced in such excess that they may even roll down the cheeks when the eyes are particularly uncomfortable. This does not do any good, though, since the tears are too watery to keep the cornea well lubricated.

Until recently, sicca has usually been treated with specially thickened drops put into the eyes several times a day or even, in many cases, several times an hour. Now, a new product on the market named Lacrisert makes life much easier for all concerned. It is a tiny (one by 3.5 mm) bean-shaped disc of special cellulose which fits comfortably inside the lower eyelid and slowly dissolves over a period of 24 hours while releasing a mucus-like material that thickens the tears. Sold in sterile packages of 60 with a special applicator, this product of the Merck drug company can really be help for dry eyes.

Eyelid Dermatitis

Because the delicate skin of the eyelids is only about one quarter as thick as the skin elsewhere, it is unusually sensitive to irritants. Accordingly, it is not uncommon for the eyelids to become itchy, red, and swollen in response to an ingredient of a cosmetic that has been applied to some other part of the body. This can occur even when the primary site to which the offending substance has been applied remains entirely normal.

Thus, eyelid dermatitis is not uncommon in response to nail polish or nail varnish, face creams, makeup, hair dye, hair spray, etc. The reaction can be either an allergic one or an irritant response to traces of a substance carried to the eyelids by the fingers, the journal *Cutis* (34#216) reports. Without realizing it, most of us touch our eyelids many times a day, even if they are not causing the slightest discomfort. Determining the cause can be difficult since the skin on the part of the body used for testing may not be sufficiently sensitive. To enhance its sensitivity, "closed" testing is employed in which the potential allergen or irritant is applied to the skin under a plastic cover. This seems to be an effective way to determine what is causing the eyelid dermatitis.

Effective Sunglasses: What You Must Ask For

When buying sunglasses, look for those that filter ultraviolet (UV) light, the tumor-producing component of sunshine, and thereby block its entry to the eyes. This helps to prevent cancer of the iris, the colored tissue that surrounds the pupils. UV light is now also thought to be a causative factor in some eye diseases formerly attributed to "aging."

Thus, the *Western Journal of Medicine* (144:454) reports, the cumulative effect of UV on the retina over a period of several decades seems to be a major factor in the development of macular degeneration, one of the most common causes of failing vision, even blindness, in the elderly.

While passing through an eye, however, much of the UV in a sunlight beam gets filtered out by the lens, which, in this way, serves as a shield for the retina. Not surprisingly, therefore, the lens bears some of the brunt of repeated and prolonged exposure to UV, becoming discolored and opaque as the result. Known as cataract, this lens condition produces progressive visual clouding until all that can be sensed is the difference between darkness and light.

Fortunately, these bad effects of UV light upon the retina and lens can be prevented with sunglasses that filter UV from sunlight, thereby stopping it from even entering the eye. However, many sunglasses don't filter out enough UV light to protect us properly, even when their manufacturer states that they are "UV absorbing." By itself, that claim can be misleading since any glass or plastic blocks at least some UV.

To properly protect the eyes, we need sunglasses that block out light of all wavelengths below 400 nm (nanometers). As a rule of thumb, lenses that can do this should be dark enough not to let you see your own pupils when looking in a mirror. Glasses that merely block out UV wavelengths below 350 are not good enough. Actually, there is now an instrument that enables professionals to determine if sunglasses can absorb UV sufficiently. This is why you ought to go to an eye professional when purchasing a new pair.

Should You Buy Bifocals?

Most people with good vision first need reading glasses in their 40s or 50s. Although they can still read without spectacles, they then start holding books at arm's length to see them clearly. Thereafter, every few years, stronger glasses are needed to keep printed words comfortably in focus.

For those of us needing new spectacles, a useful tip recently appeared in the *New England Journal of Medicine* (301:1066) — don't throw away your old ones. Your first glasses, which are no longer strong enough for reading, may be just perfect for helping you to see things a few yards away, such as watching TV, etc. Keeping your old glasses can therefore save you the expense of bifocals. The expense of bifocals becomes justifiable only if your work makes it necessary for you to keep changing spectacles to see both near and far.

FIBROCYSTIC BREASTS

Vitamin E and Fibrocystic Breasts

About 20 percent of American women have fibrocystic breasts, a condition in which small tender lumps can be felt within the breasts. Composed of distorted fluid-containing milk ducts and fibrous tissue, these lumps usually become tighter and more tender at the time of menstrual periods, when they may become so painful as to interfere with sleep.

Please note that we no longer talk about fibrocystic "disease," since we now realize that this condition is merely a variant in texture of the normal breast. It is not precancerous. Nevertheless, fibrocystic breasts often become so tight and uncomfortable that many women need treatment of one kind or another to relieve the pain.

According to the *Journal of the American Medical Association* (244:1077), vitamin E may be what they are looking for. It was found that fibrocystic occurrences disappeared or decreased in 22 of 26 women who took this vitamin in doses of 600 units daily for 12 weeks. Possibly vitamin E acts as an anti-hormone, blocking the effects of the breast-stimulating hormone prolactin, which is normally produced by the pituitary gland.

Caffeine and Fibrocystic Breasts

Women with fibrocystic breasts are usually told to give up all caffeine-containing drinks, chocolate, and medications that contain caffeine.

Now, as an outcome of the latest investigation of the cause of this condition, the *Journal of the American Medical Association* (253:2388) reports, we now know that caffeine does not stir up fibrocystic breasts and has absolutely no effect, good or bad, on this condition. Prior research into the effect of caffeine on fibrocystic breasts probably gave us misleading results, since normal women were not also included in the studies as "controls." Without controls, research often gives wrong answers. So, according to the *Journal*, women with fibrocystic breasts need no longer deny themselves coffee and chocolate, etc.

FOOT PROBLEMS

Claw Nails

When a toenail is curved and so greatly thickened that it looks more like a claw, we are dealing with a condition medically known as onychogryphosis.

This nail deformity occurs, according to *Cutis* (34:480), if toenails are not trimmed often enough and are allowed to grow to too great a length. Pressure from socks and shoes on the ends of the long nails bends them downwards and exerts leverage on their roots, irritating them and causing them to produce much thicker nails than usual. Since claw nails are difficult to cut, they tend to be further neglected and become still thicker and longer. Not surprisingly, therefore, most physicians believe them to be irreversible.

A case reported in *Cutis*, however, demonstrates that claw nails can be reversed. To achieve this, the affected nails must be cut back and trimmed to relieve the nail roots of leverage. This requires professional help repeatedly. Also, until a new nail has formed, the feet must be rested most of the time.

FROSTBITE

Take These Precautions in Cold Weather

Frostbite is becoming common during cold winter weather. Fortunately, most cases are nothing more serious than "frost-nip" at the tip of the nose or the edge of an ear. Victims momentarily feel stinging pain in the involved skin, which thereafter becomes white and painless as ice crystals form in the affected tissue. Quick cure is obtained by warming the nipped skin (by touching it) right away and thereafter shielding it against the cold.

Serious frostbite is usually due to wet socks or gloves. After an initial painful coldness, there is a progressive loss of sensation. This is misleading because the victim may not complain again until stiffness and loss of function set in (when the frostbite spreads deeper to involve bones and joints). The affected skin becomes pale, hard, and pulseless as the blood in the involved arteries freezes solid, thereby locally arresting the circulation.

Serious frostbite is treated by rapid rewarming in a tub or sink. The water temperature, according to *Conn's Current Therapy*, should be kept between 38° and 40° C (100°-105°F). Make sure it is not too hot because the victim has no sensation and is easily burned. Pain pills are best given before the victim complains, because sensation will suddenly return during rewarming (two aspirins can be quite helpful).

Rewarming should be continued until the skin looks pink (it will look redder than normal), and the tissues feel soft again. This usually takes 30 to 45 minutes. Do not rub the affected part while it is being rewarmed; this only damages the skin. After rewarming, gently dab the part dry (no rubbing), cover it with sterile dressings, and keep it at rest with the fingers or toes separated with cotton or gauze. Skin blisters usually develop in a day or two and are not necessarily a bad sign. If the blister fluid becomes cloudy or bloody, however, seek medical attention right away so that antibiotics, etc., can be given.

During cold weather, older people or anyone with heart trouble, regardless of age, should keep the lower face covered with a scarf. This is very important because cold air in the lungs reflexly constricts the coronary arteries and can thereby trigger a heart attack.

HAIR LOSS AND HAIR PROBLEMS

Hair Loss

An otherwise fit young lady went to see her doctor because she had developed a band of baldness, extending from ear to ear all the way over the top of her head. From the history and examination, the physician concluded that her alopecia (the medical term for baldness) most likely resulted from the friction and pressure exerted by a pair of heavy earphones through which she listened to music while jogging. Anything that fits tightly on the head while, at the same time rubbing against it, may cause hair to be worn away at the site of frictional contact, a letter to the editor of the *Journal of the American Medical Association* (252:3367) reports. Hair regrew quickly on this young lady's head after she switched to lighter earphones.

Baldness and Beta-Blockers

Although beta-blocker drugs are used for high blood pressure and for the prevention of angina pectoris (chest pain originating in the heart) and, as a group, are now one of the most widely prescribed types of medication, it is not yet generally known that they are sometimes responsible for a considerable loss of hair.

The journal *Cutis* (35:148) reports a 62-year-old man who had always had a healthy head of hair but who, over a period of six weeks, gradually lost most of it. Shortly before this occurred, he had started taking nadolol, also known as Cor-gard, the new long-acting beta-blocker medicine. The cause-and-effect relationship between his use of this drug and the hair loss was not immediately recognized because he also had a scaly itching scalp. Since he had assumed that the itching, scaling scalp was caused by dandruff, he had treated the symptoms with a tar-containing shampoo.

Both the hair loss and this dermatitis cleared up soon after he stopped taking nadolol, so that his scalp slowly regained its normal appearance over the next three months. Hair loss, both on the scalp and body, although uncommon, has occurred with most beta-blocker drugs.

Dandruff

Dandruff, the most common cause of itchiness of the scalp and excessive shedding of scales (scurf), affects up to 70 percent of Americans from time to time, the *U. S. Pharmacist* (9:22) reports. Scalp itching and scaliness also occurs with psoriasis and seborrheic dermatitis, diseases that are much less common than dandruff and that, fortunately, are not made worse by the usual treatments for dandruff.

Although it cannot be permanently "cured" by shampoos and always comes back again from time to time, dandruff can be kept under control with these preparations. There are many of them, fortunately, and one can nearly always be found that suits the individual and works reasonably well. If you are having difficulty in controlling dandruff, tell your pharmacist which shampoos you have tried, and ask him to recommend another that might work better for you.

One point that the *U. S. Pharmacist* makes very strongly and which one cannot afford to ignore is that it is essential to follow the written directions. Many people, for instance, do not leave the shampoo on the scalp long enough to do any good before rinsing it off, or, conversely, they fail to rinse the scalp well enough to remove all traces of the medication. This is important because many anti-dandruff chemicals are so irritating when allowed to remain on the skin for too long that they themselves can cause a dandruff-like condition.

Hair Analysis

The amounts of trace elements, such as potassium, copper, or zinc, that can be detected in human hair depends not only upon their concentration in the body but also upon how quickly the hair has been growing. Thus, when illness, deficiency, or dieting temporarily slows hair growth, little potassium and almost no copper or zinc gets into the hair, even though blood levels of these elements remain within normal limits.

Hair analysis, according to correspondence in the *Lancet* (2:608), is really only useful in detecting certain substances, such as lead or arsenic, when they have been in the body in excessive amounts for some time. Hair analysis is not really capable of demonstrating transient chemical changes in the tissues, nor is it a useful tool in assessing general health or nutritional status. Many people, unfortunately, undergo hair analysis believing that it provides valuable information that cannot be obtained easily by other means.

HEADACHE

Thunderclap Headache

An intense headache of abrupt onset, the so-called "thunderclap" headache, may be the first sign of hemorrhage inside the brain, the *Lancet* (2:1247) reports. In the words of a victim of this headache, it felt as if "a hammer had hit my head." The cause is usually bleeding inside the skull.

In deciding what to do for patients with headache of this kind, the doctor needs special X-ray pictures of the skull to display the blood vessels inside the brain. The X-rays will usually show that part of one of the arteries has become inflated like a balloon. Known as an aneurysm, this sac of blood bulges out from part of an artery that has been abnormally thin-walled since birth. Pressure from the blood inside the artery gradually distends the aneurysm until, after many years, it begins to burst. When this causes sudden massive bleeding within the skull, the victim loses consciousness and is unlikely to survive.

When there is merely a small "warning" leakage of blood from an aneurysm, however, the victim remains conscious and experiences the characteristic thunderclap headache. This first bleeding, according to the *Journal of Neurosurgery* (66:35), often gives rise to severe pain that is sharply localized to one side of the head or face, or in and around one eye. People experiencing this type of pain and who do not usually have severe headaches should, if possible, be taken to a hospital right away rather than to a doctor's office, since special tests are needed to confirm the diagnosis. Every minute counts when surgery must be performed to stop bleeding inside the skull. Such victims can usually be rescued by neurosurgery, if it is not too long delayed.

Migraine Headaches

An article in *Emergency Medicine* (16#14:69) contained some rather practical ideas about preventing headaches that migraine sufferers may wish to try.

It is especially important, the article emphasized, for these people to limit their intake of caffeine because, when taken in excess, caffeine can bring on attacks. An excess of caffeine is defined as taking more than 500 mg per day, an amount that is contained in five cups of strong coffee. The need for restricting one's caffeine intake applies not only to one's coffee drinking but also to one's total caffeine intake from all sources.

Migraine sufferers must also eat very regularly, to the point that they get up for breakfast at the same time every day, even on weekends, in order to avoid hypoglycemia (low blood sugar), which can trigger migraine. For the same reason, they should always eat at regular intervals and avoid excess carbohydrates. Furthermore, they should not eat foods that are rich in tyramine (e.g., aged cheeses, chicken livers), sodium nitrate (found in cured meats), or sodium glutamate (which is widely used in prepared foods). It is also important to note that some migraine headaches are triggered by food allergies, which is the subject of the next article.

Migraine sufferers are much less tolerant of high altitudes than are normal persons and should take the drug Diamox (acetazolamine) before ascending. In addition, since they react to feminizing hormones, they should not take oral contraceptives or, after the menopause, estrogens for the prevention of osteoporosis.

Migraine and Food Allergy

Though the cause of migraine headaches remains a mystery, *Postgraduate Medicine* (75#4:221) reports that in a group of 99 children with frequent migraine, about 85 percent were relieved of their headaches after being kept on a diet containing only those substances to which almost no one ever becomes allergic. Thereafter, usual foods were added back to the diet one at a time, and in this way, it was possible to find a food that caused relapse in 90 percent of cases.

"Trigger" foods, in their descending order of importance, were cow's milk, egg, chocolate, orange, wheat, benzoic acid (a preservative), cheese, tomato, tartrazine (the food-coloring agent, "Yellow dye #5"), rye, fish, pork, beef, corn, and soy.

Since many children do not get a headache for two to seven days after exposure to the trigger foodstuff, these dietary tests are often so difficult to interpret that they are really not too helpful. The alternative method of investigation, skin testing, is also not very sensitive or reliable. For these reasons, it is often better to go ahead and try a diet that is free of all known trigger foods, without even attempting to discover which one (or ones) is causing the trouble.

Ice Packs for Headache

Victims of migraine and other frequent headaches rarely obtain complete relief with medication. Well aware of this, researchers at Chicago's Diamond Headache Clinic have been trying to help by cooling patients' heads with ice.

Actually, rather than ice, they use gel packs (trade name Cold Comfort) that are sold by drug stores for the treatment of sprains. These gel packs remain soft and can be molded to fit body contours even after they are frozen. About 75 percent of headache victims found this treatment to be effective and intend to continue using it. Migraine, incidentally, was by far the most responsive type of headache, *Postgraduate Medicine* (79#1:305) reports.

HEART ATTACKS

A Silent Warning of Heart Attack

When the amount of blood flowing through the coronary arteries is less than the heart muscle needs (a situation known as ischemia), one commonly experiences a tight, crushing sensation or pain (angina pectoris) in the center of the chest, or sometimes elsewhere (e.g., the left arm).

Only rarely, it has been customarily believed, does ischemia occur without anginal pain, a situation known as silent ischemia. Now, however, the *New England Journal of Medicine* (318:1005) reports, it has been discovered that silent ischemia occurs quite often, especially at times of mental stress. Stress causes ischemia by temporarily constricting the blood vessels of the heart.

Another finding of this research is that many people at different times have both types of ischemia (i.e., either the painful or the silent kind). Thus, if with treatment a patient experiences less anginal pain, it cannot be assumed that his condition is improved. He might just be having silent ischemia instead. Reduction of anginal symptoms, therefore, can no longer be relied upon as a guide to the amount of physical or mentally stressful activity in which heart disease victims can engage.

Fortunately, an editorial in the *Journal* (318:1058) points out, we can still gauge a heart's degree of ischemic impairment (or lack thereof) by studying its electrical tracings on a continuous 24-hour EKG. Such monitoring can be performed as the person goes about his normal activities while wearing a small device (Holter monitor) about the size of a Walkman radio. Actually, this type of monitoring is a better guide to the heart's condition and need for treatment than are the patient's symptoms.

If coronary heart disease is suspected, therefore, be sure to visit your doctor regularly for monitoring, even if you have no anginal pain.

Heart Attacks and Exercise

Sudden death from heart attack is two to three times more likely to occur in the morning than at any other time of day, the *Boston Globe* reports. Harvard researchers think this is linked with a daily surge in the blood clotting mechanism that is at its height early in the day.

This tendency toward clotting is particularly dangerous for people whose coronary arteries (the vessels that feed the heart muscle) have become narrowed by deposits of cholesterol. The combination of blood clots and a partly blocked artery is a bad one that can too easily result in a complete stoppage of blood flow.

The big question, then, according to the *Physician and*

Sportsmedicine (15#4:39), is whether coronary heart disease patients should avoid taking exercise in the mornings. Obviously, the answer is "Yes." It is probably safer for them to exercise later in the day. Even more importantly, however, they should recognize the warning symptoms of a threatened heart attack and stop exercising, at any time of day, when any of these are present. Tiredness, breathlessness, pain or a sensation of tightness in the chest, neck, or in the left arm are the most common warning signs. In addition, of course, they should go to see a doctor right away.

Self-Administered Resuscitation

The life of a heart attack victim who collapses in public can often be saved by an onlooker who knows how to give CPR (cardiopulmonary resuscitation). In CPR, mouth-to-mouth breathing pushes oxygen into the lungs while rhythmical pressure over the heart maintains the circulation. Without this, permanent brain damage or death would result in four to six minutes.

Those who have heart attacks when alone are in much greater danger. Without help, the person whose heart stops beating properly and who begins to feel faint has only about 10 seconds left before he loses consciousness.

According to *Emergency Medicine*, however, heart attack victims can help themselves by repeated coughing. A very deep breath must be taken before each cough, and the cough must be strong and prolonged, as in producing sputum from deep inside the chest. A breath and a cough must be repeated every one to two seconds without letup until help arrives or until the heart is felt to be beating normally again.

Deep breaths get oxygen into the lungs, and coughing

movements squeeze the heart and keep the blood circulating. In this way, heart attack victims can get to a telephone and, between breaths, call for help.

Aspirin and Heart Attacks

Although much has been written about the use of aspirin to reduce the likelihood of a heart attack due to blockage of a coronary artery — or acute myocardial infarction (AMI) — not all physicians accept it as a valid means of prevention.

Possibly explaining this lack of agreement, researchers in blood clotting have shown that aspirin in very small doses (about one five-grain tablet every other day) slows blood clotting sufficiently to help prevent heart attacks, but that the large (eight tablets) daily doses tried by most cardiologists make blood clotting more likely.

Now, in addition, according to the American *Journal of Cardiology* (47:1210), Japanese cardiologists have found that certain persons who are prone to angina pectoris (chest pain due to coronary artery spasm) actually experience angina more often when taking large doses of aspirin. These people then also have a weaker than normal heartbeat during exercise, with abnormal heart tracings (EKG).

In view of these findings, if you are heart attack prone, it would be a good idea to avoid taking aspirin regularly in large doses.

Nitroglycerin and Heart Attacks

Nitroglycerin, held under the tongue or rubbed on the skin, is an established drug for angina pectoris, the chest pain that afflicts people with narrowed coronary arteries. Angina occurs whenever too little blood reaches the myocardium (heart muscle) to meet its demands in response to exercise or emotion. Nitroglycerin relaxes arteries generally, thereby removing any coronary spasm contributing to angina. Nitroglycerin's drawback is that it also lowers the blood pressure (BP), and since the BP falls during heart attacks anyway, lowering it still further could be dangerous. This is why doctors used to stop the drug during heart attacks.

Nowadays, according to the *American Journal of Cardiology* (49:842), doctors are beginning to use nitroglycerin to improve myocardial blood flow during heart attacks. They manage to do this safely by keeping their patients lying down with their legs elevated while nitroglycerin is employed. This prevents blood from flowing away from the heart and into the legs by gravity. Patients whose symptoms suddenly worsen (possibly owing to a heart attack) after they have taken nitroglycerin should therefore lie down and put their legs up. About the worst thing they could do would be to drive themselves to the hospital. Rather, they should go by ambulance, or lie down in the back of the car, and let somebody else do the driving.

Here's another warning: A doctor writing in the *New England Journal of Medicine* (308:782) reports that a heart patient who urgently needed an NTG tablet died while struggling to get one out of a previously unopened bottle. Fatal delay occurred while the patient tried to pull the cotton stuffing out of the bottle. To avoid this danger, all patients who rely upon sublingual NTG are advised to open their new bottles of this medicine while a few tablets still remain instantly available in another container.

Alcohol and Heart Attacks

The notion that moderate drinking helps to prevent death from heart attack has been considerably strengthened by a 10-year study in California involving people who routinely visited Kaiser-Permanente Hospitals for annual check-ups.

The lowest mortality in these people, according to the *British Medical Journal* (284:444), was among those consuming one or two alcoholic drinks a day. Taking their heart attack death rate as 1.0, the rate for teetotalers was 1.5 (50 percent higher). The rate for people taking three to five drinks daily was also 1.5. For still heavier drinkers, the rate was two. Three other studies (two in the U.S., one in England) have shown the same sort of U-shaped curve relating mortality rates with alcohol consumed.

However, further study has revealed that those who drink moderately need to be divided into two groups. Group 1 appears to benefit from moderate drinking. These people, according to the *Journal of Cardiovascular Medicine* (6:309) have a good blood supply to their heart muscle. Persons in Group 2, a majority among moderate drinkers, have one or more narrowed coronary arteries and have a higher than usual incidence of coronary heart attack.

The difference in alcohol's effect, it appears, depends upon its ability to increase blood flow through the coronary arteries by dilating them. When the coronaries are normal, alcohol therefore increases all of the heart muscle's blood supply. In people who have a coronary artery which has become narrowed and rigid by atherosclerosis, blood flow is further reduced in the narrow vessel at times when flow is being increased in the healthy wider vessels. This happens because blood always flows along the path of least resistance and is therefore selectively diverted away from narrow vessels when the normal ones open up more widely. Known as the "Coronary Steal Syndrome," this diversion of blood away from certain vessels can bring on a heart attack.

It is clear, therefore, that people who have angina pectoris (pain or tightness in the chest during exercise due to a narrow coronary) should avoid alcohol entirely.

Magnesium and Heart Attacks

There is a strong association between the incidence of cardiovascular disease (hardened arteries, hypertension, and heart attacks) and soft drinking water. This association, however, is not perfect, and there are just enough soft water districts with low heart disease rates to make it obvious that we don't yet have the whole story.

One possible explanation is that magnesium (which can be present in soft water) has also recently been found to protect against cardiovascular disease. According to the *Western Journal of Medicine* (133:304), calcium and magnesium both act in the intestine by combining with dietary fat to form insoluble soap-like compounds that are not absorbed, thereby limiting the amount of fat entering the bloodstream. About two mg of magnesium per pound of body weight daily is optimal, the *Western Journal* reports.

Ice Water and the Heart

Before reaching the stomach, swallowed food and fluid must pass down the esophagus, a tube-like structure that runs through the chest behind the heart. Because there is such a large area of contact between the esophagus and the heart, the temperature of swallowed foods is quickly conveyed to the heart, an effect that is even more pronounced when the heart is enlarged as the result of disease.

For this reason, according to the *Annals of Internal Medicine* (96:614), drinking ice water can induce serious abnormalities of the heart rhythm. It seems reasonable, therefore, to suggest that anyone with a heart ailment should be on the lookout for problems of this kind. If drinking hot or cold fluids disturbs the rate or rhythm of the heart beat, medical help is needed right away before more serious harm results.

Wrinkled Ear Lobes and Liability to Heart Attack

Much has been written recently about the relationship between deep wrinkles in the skin of the ear lobes (running obliquely upwards from front to back) and increased liability to heart attacks. Many cardiologists find this a valuable sign for detecting people who are at greater than normal risk. Other heart specialists are not so impressed and believe that ear lobe creases merely reflect aging and obesity, both of which are associated with higher than average heart attack rates.

Now that the medical profession has had more time to look into the matter, we can say that, although conflicting, both opinions are right. It depends on the population studied. Finns, according to *Lancet*, have a high (90 percent) correlation between ear lobe creases and coronary heart disease, while Hawaiians of Japanese ancestry often have ear creases without coronary heart disease.

It seems advisable, therefore, for any Caucasian with ear lobe creases to have a checkup by a cardiologist. Even if no heart problem is discovered, it will be comforting to know that the odds are in your favor.

Hairy Ears and Heart Disease

Along the same lines as the previous article, this one is prompted by a letter written to the editor of the *New England Journal of Medicine* (311:1317) from a group of physicians in New York, who suggest that hairy ears, with bristles growing out from the ear canals as well as upon the external parts of the ears, may be another sign of coronary proneness.

They admit, however, that ear hairiness is a male trait. It is already known that the longer men live, the hairier their noses and ears become. In addition, of course, the older a man is, the more likely he is to have developed hardened arteries (atherosclerosis) and coronary heart disease. Perhaps, therefore, hairiness of the ears is not any better as a coronary heart disease predictor than is the smoking of pipes by wearers of trousers, both of which habits (together) are more prevalent in older men. Associations can fool us if we become overawed by statistics.

HEARTBURN

Sleeping Pills and Heartburn

When there is an excess of acid in the stomach, some of it may be regurgitated back into the throat, thereby producing a strong acid taste in the mouth known as heartburn. When heartburn keeps one awake at night, *Geriatrics* (41#1:31) reports, taking a sleeping pill is not a safe thing to do.

The pill will overcome the insomnia, but it can also prevent a heartburn victim from waking up in response to the discomfort of the acid regurgitation. If acid is allowed to remain in the esophagus (the passageway through which food and drink descend from the throat to the stomach) for any length of time without being neutralized with milk or medication, it will erode the lining of the esophagus The entire thickness of the esophageal wall will become inflamed and go into spasms, a very painful condition known as reflux esophagitis. Without a sleeping pill, the victim is likely to be aroused by the discomfort of heartburn and to take steps to relieve it before it can do any harm.

Antacids' Effects on Medication

Except for their slightly constipating effect, antacids are bland and do not cause side effects, at least not immediately. The aluminum-containing antacids, however, may have some undesirable effects on the bones and brain that only show up much later on in life. But even calcium antacids, such as calcium carbonate (the principle ingredient of Tums), which are ordinarily completely safe, are not entirely harmless, according to the *Consumers Union News Digest* (11:23:9), since they can alter the effects of other medications taken at the same time.

Antacids speed absorption of certain drugs, thereby possibly producing symptoms of overdosage that, in some cases, could be dangerous. Absorption of certain other drugs is delayed by antacids, and this could result in reduced effectiveness. In view of these potential interactions, therefore, anyone who is taking a prescription drug should check with a physician or pharmacist before starting to take an antacid as well.

HEART PROBLEMS

Early Warning of Heart Failure

Depending on the type of heart trouble, some of the earliest signs of failure in need of treatment include swelling of the ankles (medically known as edema) and shortness of breath during mild exercise, such as climbing stairs. This latter sign is evidence that the heart is not pumping well enough to empty blood out of the lungs, causing the condition medically known as pulmonary congestion.

However, according to *Primary Cardiology Clinics* (2#1:19), a certain type of coughing is yet another sign that, if heeded, gives even earlier warning. Also due to pulmonary congestion, this sign is almost like a smoker's "hacking" cough. Its really distinctive feature is that it comes on when one is in bed or sitting down but stops almost instantly when one stands up.

In heart failure patients, this sign may precede breathlessness by hours or days but should always be reported to a physician right away. When pulmonary congestion is more severe, of course, the cough is not relieved by standing and may be replaced by breathlessness which is not relieved by rest. Even though this early sign is not new, we feel that knowing about it is important and could save many lives.

Side Effects of Digitalis

Digitalis, the historic heart medicine extracted from the foxglove plant, and modern drugs chemically related to it (e.g: Digoxin) are often taken by people with heart failure for the rest of their lives. Under these circumstances, unfortunately, dangerous amounts of digitalis may slowly accumulate in the tissues. This can occur so slowly that "patients treated with digitalis in the long term may creep quietly into a semi-intoxicated state after, say, 10 to 15 years," a cardiologist quoted by *Modern Medicine* (52#12:55) reports. To avoid this danger, those taking digitalis for a long time must be assessed by their physicians periodically to determine if the dosage should be reduced or discontinued.

Commonly recognized digitalis side effects include nausea, vomiting, irregular or slow pulse, low blood pressure, diarrhea, and yellow vision. More recently, according to the *British Medical Journal* (284:162), epileptic seizures have been recognized as digitalis-induced. Nervous system effects of digitalis also include headache, confusion, weakness, drowsiness, and psychosis. Symptoms such as these are often ascribed to hardening of the arteries or a "minor stroke." Since so many older people take digitalis, we must be careful not to overlook these drug effects.

The latest on this topic, according to *Emergency Medicine* (19#11:114) is that, most commonly, the first symptom of digitalis intoxication is a stomach upset, which is often attributed to something else. The usual story is that a heart failure patient has been taking one of these drugs without difficulty for several months, or even for years, and then begins to complain of nausea, lack of appetite, occasional vomiting, and (less commonly) diarrhea.

To avoid these toxic cumulative effects, some doctors give their patients occasional "holidays" from treatment with the drug, omitting dosage entirely for one day (usually on a Sunday, when there is less stress on the heart) every week. In this way, their patients can "spill off" any slight excess of the drug that has started to accumulate. However, patients on heart drugs should not decide to make changes in dosage for themselves, even when new symptoms occur, but should consult a doctor first.

Propranolol and Breathing

Propranolol, the beta-blocker drug that is very often used, among many things, for the treatment of high blood pressure and various heart conditions, has been found to exert a profoundly weakening effect on the muscles of respiration and especially on the diaphragm. In this respect it is just about as different from theophylline as it could be .

According to the *American Family Physician* (30#1:225), this weakening effect decreases the amount of air that can be moved in and out of the lungs with each breath by about 15 percent, a reduction that is more than enough to endanger a person who, for any reason, already has some difficulty in breathing. Thus, people with breathlessness due to COPD, heart failure, asthma, etc., could slip into an even worse state of respiratory distress if they receive a medication such as propranolol.

Heart Pain at Night

Raising up the head of one's bed so as to tilt its foot downwards by 10 degrees helps reduce the likelihood of angina pectoris (pain the in the chest due to heart disease) occurring at night, *Geriatrics* (40#3:23) reports. It works by allowing more blood to pool by gravity into the legs, thereby taking the strain off an overloaded heart. An alternative, of course, is to take a long-acting medication, such as nitroglycerin on the skin, which relaxes the blood vessels and thereby diverts blood away from the heart in much the same way. Preventing anginal pain with blocks under the bed (10 inches high) rather than with drugs, of course, is much safer since there are no side effects. See the article, "Nitroglycerin and Heart Attacks."

Blood Clotting and Tonic Water

Spontaneous clotting of blood in the circulation will cause a stroke (if the clot lodges in one of the brain's blood vessels) or a heart attack (if it blocks one of the heart's coronary arteries). To prevent recurrences, many people recovering from a stroke or a heart attack are given daily doses of one of the anticoagulant drugs, such as Warfarin or Coumadin. Other conditions, too, (e.g., heart valve abnormalities) may require long-term anticoagulation. Since too much drug will result in bleeding, and too little of it provides no benefit at all, regular testing is required to make sure that the patient's dosage needs are being exactly met.

Change in dosage requirement could occur in anyone who drinks tonic water, a major ingredient of which is quinine. Quinine, reports the *British Medical Journal* (286:1258), interacts with anticoagulants, making their effect more powerful. Anticoagulant users, therefore, should be careful to avoid any drinks that are made with tonic water.

How Safe Is Caffeine for People with Heart Disease?

Although there is no evidence that coffee brings on heart attacks, it is well-known that drinking too much coffee or other caffeine-containing beverages makes the heart beat faster and drives up the blood pressure. Not so well known is that fact that, depending on the dosage, caffeine may have exactly opposite effects on the heart and blood vessels.

In small doses, according to the *British Medical Journal* (2:28), caffeine's excitatory effects on the cardiovascular system are usually countered by its effect on the brain and nerves, which then relay slowing and calming signals to the heart and blood vessels. At higher doses, caffeine's excitatory effects on the cardiovascular system overcome its calming effects from the brain. For people with heart disease, therefore, it is best not to take that second cup.

Aspirin and Surgery

Many people now take a small dose of aspirin every day or every second day to lessen their chances of getting a coronary heart attack. Aspirin helps them to do this by rendering their blood less capable of clotting (during most heart attacks, an artery in the heart that has become narrowed by deposits of cholesterol becomes completely blocked off by a clot of blood).

However, no drug, including aspirin, is without side effects of some sort, and in this case we need to be concerned that loss of clotting ability could be dangerous during surgery. In fact, *Emergency Medicine* (19#18:57) points out that aspirin significantly increases the incidence of complications due to blood loss after such procedures as tooth extraction, facial plastic surgery, tonsillectomy, and coronary artery bypass graft operations. Although less noticeable, this effect of aspirin could mar the result of any operation. Adequate clotting, of course, is necessary to seal off and stop oozing from blood vessels that are cut across during operations, even though they have been tied off by the surgeon.

To reduce this risk of postoperative bleeding as much as possible, aspirin should be discontinued for at least a week before surgery. When this is not possible, be sure the surgeon knows if you have been taking aspirin. He can then test the blood and decide whether something needs to be done to restore clotting to normal before he operates. Other medications that interfere with clotting include non-steroidal anti-inflammatory drugs (NSAIDs) such as Advil, Clinoril, Feldene, Indocin, Motrin, Nalfon, Naprosyn, Nuprin, and Tolectin, which are used for arthritic pain, headache, and menstrual cramps, etc. Fish oil products, such as Maxepa, and vitamin E can do the same thing. Since several other drugs also have this effect, be sure to tell the surgeon about every medication that you are taking.

Fish and Heart Disease

One issue of the *New England Journal of Medicine* (312:1205) contains three papers and an editorial that are concerned with the effects of fish-eating and coronary heart disease.

As previously reported, the unsaturated fatty acids in fish benefit mankind by reducing the amount of atherosclerosis (narrowing of the arteries by deposits of cholesterol) and thereby preserving an adequate blood flow through the coronary arteries that supply the muscle of the heart.

One of the papers reports a study involving 852 Dutchmen, whose health and diets were studied for over 20 years. The incidence of death from coronary heart disease was over 50 percent lower among those who consumed at least 30 grams (about one ounce) of fish every day than it was among those who ate none at all. It was found, furthermore, that some benefit is obtained even when fish dishes are eaten only twice a week.

HEMORRHOIDS

Bleeding Hemorrhoids

In addition to causing pain, hemorrhoids can bleed enough to produce anemia, which, in turn, may put enough strain upon an elderly person's heart to throw it into failure, *Geriatrics* (39#8:89) reports. In younger people whose hearts are stronger, this anemia may nevertheless help to cause angina (pain or a feeling of tightness in the chest, originating in the heart, and brought on by exercise or emotion).

When an elderly person has both heart failure and bleeding hemorrhoids, it can be dangerous to stop the bleeding by conventional means since such patients cannot easily withstand an anesthetic or the trauma of surgery. Now, however, with the new and much safer procedure known as cryosurgery, which involves freezing the unwanted tissues with an extremely cold (minus 70 degrees C) nitrous oxide probe, the risk has virtually been eliminated. Patients treated in this way rarely require anesthesia and are free of pain immediately after the procedure. Cryosurgery is safely performed in a doctor's office, and has even been used successfully in 80-year-olds with heart failure caused by massive rectal bleeding. Since cryosurgery destroys any sensory nerves frozen by the probe, the postoperative course is painless. Not yet available widely, cryosurgery should catch on very quickly if this initial experience can be confirmed.

HIATUS HERNIA

Living with Hiatus Hernia

Food, drink and gastric acid are normally prevented from backing up into the esophagus by a ring of muscle that encircles the top of the stomach. This mechanism fails in the condition known as hiatus hernia, resulting in a permanent liability to inflammation of the esophagus by gastric acid, a painful complication known as esophagitis.

Writing in the *Lancet* (1:158) about his personal experience with hiatus hernia, a physician stresses the need to remain upright after every meal and never to bend over, even momentarily, until the stomach's contents have moved on into the intestine. One learns by experience when this occurs. Although it is easy to remain upright during the day, it is much more difficult to do so when asleep at night. Never take a sedative in the hope of sleeping through the discomfort that will result from lying down too soon after a late meal. Under these circumstances, the physician has found, it is better to sit up half the night, if necessary, until the meal has settled. Better yet, he suggests, avoid late meals entirely.

HERPES

Herpes in Hot Tubs

Several health spas were recently closed down for a short time when some of their patrons complained about developing genital herpes after using their facilities. Public health workers investigated those spas but failed to demonstrate any herpes virus in the water of their hot tubs, on benches, or elsewhere, the *Journal of the American Medical Association* (250:3081) reports.

Nevertheless, the report continues, they were able to show that live herpes virus can survive on plastic and tiled surfaces that are kept warm and moist. Conceivably, then, scantily clad or nude patrons who have genital herpes could contaminate surfaces in a steam room, hot tub, or pool area, thereby infecting others who sit in the same place soon afterwards. Since the hot tubs and pools of spas are known to be responsible for the spread of other infections, such as conjunctivitis and boils, there is some reason to be concerned. Nevertheless, the Journal report concludes, it is unlikely that genital herpes spreads in the same way since the virus probably needs to be frictionally rubbed into the skin or onto a mucosal surface before it can take hold sufficiently to produce an infection, if that is any comfort.

HICCUPS

Hiccups, Another Cure

Holding the breath is usually the first thing that people try for hiccups, and then they try drinking cold water. But, according to *Emergency Medicine* (17#10:152), best results are obtained when both of these methods are combined. Between hiccups, the hiccups victim should take in a very deep breath, hold it for a second, and then breathe out in order to empty the chest of air as completely as possible. Next, while still in exhalation, one should swallow a glass of water and thereafter maintain the exhalation for several seconds more.

HORMONES

Should Women Take Estrogens to Prevent Osteoporosis?

Osteoporosis (calcium loss from the bones, with fragility and increased liability to fracture) accounts for over 90,000 hip fractures in postmenopausal women every year. In addition to hip fracture, osteoporosis causes pain and disability from softening and collapse of vertebrae (spinal bones), with loss of height and rounding of the back. (See the section of this book that has been devoted to articles on this very serious disease.)

Osteoporosis, according to *Geriatrics* (37#3:18), is essentially preventable in women after the menopause if, in addition to taking calcium and vitamin D and regular exercise, they are given estrogens to replace the hormones that were produced by their ovaries before the menopause. While none of these measures must be overdone, all of them contribute to skeletal strength. Knowing this, the physician quoted by *Geriatrics* states that he finds it appalling that we are permitting this "preventable and treatable disease (osteoporosis) to blossom without doing anything about it."

The reason, of course, is that estrogens have been linked to cancer of the uterus, thereby possibly doing more harm than good. About 10 years ago, when more cases of cancer of the endometrium (lining of the womb) were being detected in menopausal women, it was thought that estrogens might be the cause. Routine estrogen treatment of older women was therefore discontinued. The thought that estrogens might have been responsible was also strengthened when it was noticed that the number of cases of endometrial cancer being detected recently fell coincident in time with reduced estrogen usage.

Giving thought to this matter, *Science* points out that the apparent increase in endometrial cancer that accompanied the widespread use of estrogen could have been due simply to better cancer detection. Improved cancer-finding may well have temporarily increased the number of cases reported, but after those cases were found, the number reported would naturally decline to the previous level.

The point seems to be well taken. If estrogens were cancer-producing, one would expect endometrial cancer to be most common before the menopause, at a time of life when estrogen concentration in a woman's body is at its highest. This is not the case.

A Mayo Clinic specialist, writing in *Geriatrics* (37#3:79), notes that estrogen treatment does not increase the risk of heart attack or breast cancer in postmenopausal women. However, the author agrees that estrogen replacement therapy does slightly increase the risk of uterine cancer. Nevertheless, the article points out, if postmenopausal women being treated with estrogens are examined regularly and understand that they must report immediately if they develop vaginal bleeding, the relatively small risk from uterine cancer (which can be caught early and treated by surgery) will be well below that from osteoporotic fractures. It is important to remember that deaths from hip fracture and its complications are five times more common than cancer of the uterus.

One other caution for women taking estrogens: If you are taking estrogens with other ovarian-type hormones in mixtures such as Amen, Curretab, or Provera, you should stop the medication and contact your physician immediately if you develop any swelling or tenderness of the breasts.

With these safeguards, according to *Geriatrics* , it seems safer for women to take estrogens after the menopause to prevent osteoporosis than to try doing without them.

Shift Work and Hormones

Shift workers are 30 percent more prone to be injured at work than are people who always work during the day, *Medical World News* (28#15:22) reports. Typically, their coffee intake is rather heavy, and they often have stomach and intestinal complaints. Changing shifts not only interferes with sleep but also changes the times of day at which the hormones (e.g., adrenalin, thyroid) are most plentiful.

The trouble is that hormone production cannot change

suddenly and can only adjust by about one hour each day. This inability of hormone blood levels to peak in synchrony with changed hours is also the basis for jet lag (see the article, "Jet Lag Explained" under the heading Insomnia and Sleep Problems). For workers who change shifts, rotations should preferably last two weeks, and if possible, changes should involve moving forward in time (like traveling westward) so that one goes to bed later rather than earlier. Also, since certain medicines interact with hormones, people with diabetes, hypertension, epilepsy, asthma, etc., should try to avoid shift work entirely.

HYPERTHYROIDISM

Hyperthyroidism and Aspirin

People being treated for hyperthyroidism (an excessively active thyroid gland) may do well for many years but then suddenly become ill with high fever, rapid bounding pulse, and extreme agitation (even mania). Known as a thyroid storm, this emergency must be dealt with in a hospital right away.

Thyroid storm can have many causes, including too much pressure on the gland during physical examination, and excessive iodine intake. Aspirin, too, according to *Emergency Medicine* (14#3:26), can trigger this emergency because it displaces thyroid hormone into the bloodstream from the tissues. Aspirin, therefore should never be given to people with hyperthyroidism. For headache and fever, etc., people with thyroid trouble can use acetaminophen in place of aspirin.

HYPOGLYCEMIA

Hypoglycemia Can Be Misdiagnosed

"Hypoglycemia" means that the concentration of sugar in the blood has fallen to less than 45 mg per 100 cc. Blood sugar levels this low adversely affect the brain, causing jitteriness, weakness, lightheadedness, bizarre behavior, episodes of memory loss, and if the hypoglycemia is sufficiently severe and long-lasting, convulsions, brain damage, coma, and even death.

Since we are all occasionally tired and forgetful, hypoglycemia tends to be diagnosed too often in people who do not really have low blood sugar concentrations, the *Mayo Clinic Proceedings* (60:844) reports. This is potentially very dangerous because overdiagnosing hypoglycemia may result in some other more serious condition being overlooked. Thus, in order to be certain of the diagnosis, the doctor must obtain a sample of blood from the patient and demonstrate that the blood sugar is low at a time when there are appropriate symptoms. He must also be able to abolish the symptoms by giving the patient sugar.

Hypoglycemia has many possible causes. "Mild" cases, which can be quickly corrected with a sugary drink, occur an hour or so after alcoholic drinks or certain medications (especially sulfa-containing ones), or in some people, even after food. "Severe" cases, which are not so easy to correct, may be due to tumors of the liver or pancreas, diabetes, or other serious illness. It is therefore important for the doctor to find out the exact cause in every case. Only in this way can he make sure that a serious disease (e.g., cancer) that needs treatment without delay is not being overlooked.

Hypoglycemia and Car Accidents

Now that diabetics are being taught to keep their blood sugar levels under tighter control with more frequent injections of regular insulin, the *American Family Physician* (30#4:189) reports, more car accidents are occurring as a result of hypoglycemia, an excessively low blood sugar level.

The nonwarning type of hypoglycemia is the most dangerous since it occurs suddenly and without the usual premonitory symptoms, such as hunger, faintness, sweating, tremor, etc. Without warning, the diabetic person begins behaving in a robot-like, purposeless manner and may convulse and lose consciousness. Many people who have had such reactions while driving have made U-turns and crashed head-on at high speed into the oncoming traffic. Medications (such as aspirin, sulfa-drugs, phenylbutazone, and beta-blockers) and alcohol make such reactions much more likely to occur.

To minimize the possibility of hypoglycemia while driving, diabetics can check their own blood sugar levels at home with a Glucometer, which is reported to be more accurate than Chemstrips. If the glucose level is below 200 mg, the situation can be quickly dealt with by taking a sugary drink and some food. On long trips, it is recommended that diabetics test the blood sugar every two hours, even if they are feeling well.

INFECTIONS FROM PETS

Infection from Dogs and Cats

Attacks of sore throat that keep coming back in spite of being treated thoroughly and repeatedly with antibiotics may be due to reinfection with bacteria that are being carried in the throat of a household pet. According to a doctor quoted by the *American Family Physician* (27#2:373), the offending bacteria living in the throats of cats and dogs are Group A hemolytic streptococci, one of the most frequent causes of acute sore throat and febrile illness in man. Complications of this infection in humans include scarlet fever, rheumatic fever, and nephritis.

Forty percent of the time when the doctor suspected reinfection by a pet and asked a veterinarian to culture its throat, the result was positive. Following treatment of the animal (with an antibiotic), no involved family had a recurrent or persistent streptococcal sore throat.

Cat Bites

Even though a cat bite looks clean, and one has washed it and applied an antiseptic, the chances are that wound sepsis will develop if an antibiotic is not given to prevent it, the *Annals of Emergency Medicine* (13:155) reports. Eleven adults with deep cat bites that appeared clean were given either an antibiotic capsule (Oxacillin 500 mg) or an identically appearing capsule of placebo four times daily for five days. Whereas five of the six on placebo developed wound infections, none of the five who got the antibiotic had any further trouble. Since cat bites have resulted in some very serious infections, including even Plague in southwestern states, be sure to report them all to your doctor.

Heartworm from Dog to Man

A report in Radiology tells of several patients with coin-sized round shadows in their chest X-rays. In each case, surgery was undertaken for suspected lung cancer, but under the microscope, none of the removed tissues proved to be cancerous, and all were found to consist of inflammatory tissues surrounding dead heartworms.

Heartworm is usually fatal to dogs, but the vast majority of human cases have no illness and go undetected. Mosquitoes convey the parasite from dog to man. In nearly every infected person, the immune defense system kills the heartworms so quickly that they don't get past the skin. In rare cases, they survive a little longer and reach the lungs, where they finally become surrounded and killed by antibodies and white blood cells. This gives rise to an irritable cough lasting several days, during which chest X-rays will temporarily show a round tumor-like mass in the lung.

Left untreated, human heartworm patients do well. However, if found to have a tumor-like chest X-ray shadow, they must undergo lung surgery to make sure it is not a cancer. It should be reemphasized that very nearly everyone who gets bitten by heartworm-infected mosquitoes quickly destroys the parasites in the skin and suffers no illness. Also, getting rid of your dog will not help in the slightest because infected mosquitoes can carry heartworm parasites clear across town. So, dog lovers, don't worry.

Getting Insects out of Ears

There is nothing like having a live insect buzzing around inside one's ear. Reflexly, one pokes at it and turns the ear downward with the hope that it will fall out, measures which merely make it struggle more. The quickest and least traumatic way of getting bugs out of ears, according to the Journal of the American Medical Association, is to float them out. Turn the occupied ear uppermost and then pour water or mineral oil into the ear canal.

INFERTILITY

Infertility and Vitamin C

When married couples try but fail to have children, both the wife and husband need to be tested. There are several possible causes. In men, the *Journal of the American Medical Association* (249:2947) reports, perhaps the easiest type of infertility to treat is caused by a deficiency of vitamin C. This vitamin is also known as ascorbic acid, a name reflecting its ability to prevent scurvy (a disabling illness, with painful bruising around the bones that used to afflict sailors after months at sea without fresh fruit or vegetables).

A much less severe vitamin C deficiency, which is by no means severe enough to produce scurvy, can cause male infertility due to clumping together of the spermatozoa. Failure of separation prevents sperm from swimming towards the ovum. Mild deficiencies of this nature are diagnosed by measuring the concentration of vitamin C in the blood. The infertility can easily be overcome in a few weeks with one or two tablets of vitamin C (500 mg each) taken every day by mouth.

Infertility from Jogging

By jogging nearly every day, two young women kept themselves very fit but were unable to become pregnant. Since neither woman had menstruated for over 12 months, both were treated with Clomiphene, a medication which induces the ovaries to start working again. Surprisingly, even in double doses, this failed to help.

As a last resort, and with some difficulty, they were persuaded to give up jogging. After just one more missed period, both women promptly became pregnant as soon as their ovarian function returned. Summarizing these cases in the *Lancet* (306:50), a gynecologist suggests that vigorous exercise is often overlooked as the cause of infertility.

INSOMNIA AND SLEEP PROBLEMS

Treating Sleep Apnea

Sleep apnea is the condition in which people frequently stop breathing at night for a disturbingly long time. Each episode ends in a burst of snoring. Because this occurs many times a night, it can interfere significantly with the brain's oxygen supply and result in morning headaches, drowsiness, and the need for many naps during the day. Ultimately, high blood pressure, heart failure, and intellectual deterioration may supervene.

This condition is due to laxity and flabbiness of tissues at the back of the throat. When the person is sleeping, this allows the tongue to fall back into the throat and cause choking. A surefire way of curing sleep apnea is to operate and create a false opening into the windpipe (tracheotomy) below the site of blockage. This, however, is disfiguring and renders the patient more than usually prone to serious chest infection.

In a safer operation, loose, redundant tissue at the back of the throat, including the tonsils and part of the soft palate, are removed, making the upper airway larger and not so prone to become blocked during sleep. A recent article in the *Archives of Internal Medicine* (141:990) supports this method of treating sleep apnea, citing a marked reduction in the number of episodes of sleep apnea that have been reported in adults whose enlarged tonsils were removed.

However, this is a painful operation and every effort should first be made to help the sleep apnea victim by non-operative means. One easy way of doing so is described in the *Southern Medical Journal* (79:1061). It points out that sleep apnea is like ordinary snoring in that it is unlikely to occur unless the victim sleeps on his back. The trick, then, is to keep the sleeper on his side and stop him from rolling onto his back. This can often be done by sewing a tennis ball onto the back of the victim's pajama jacket.

One other point to make on the subject of sleep apnea is that sedatives and alcohol tend to aggravate the problem. Therefore avoidance of sedatives and alcohol is important if you are treating this problem.

Caffeine and Insomnia

Caffeine, the coffee and tea component that wakes you up, is also to be found in over 100 widely available nonprescription drugs and in more than 65 other types of drug that doctors commonly prescribe, *Modern Medicine* (52#8:145) reports.

Accordingly, people who suffer from insomnia should read the labels on their medications to see if they contain caffeine, and ask the pharmacist or doctor, if necessary, to give them an alternative that is caffeine-free. Sometimes, however, caffeine is needed in certain combination drugs to enhance the effect of another ingredient. Lastly, many people do not realize that cocoa, chocolate, Pepsi, Coca-Cola, Tab, RC Cola, Mountain Dew, Dr Pepper, and some other soft drinks also contain a lot of caffeine.

Mercifully, most of us can take these drinks and moderate amounts of coffee without suffering from insomnia, and find that they decrease fatigue and provide a sense of well-being. Those who suffer from insomnia, however, should take caffeine-containing beverages only with breakfast and lunch and, thereafter, should avoid all sources of caffeine for the rest of the day.

Broken Sleep and the Elderly

About 70 percent of the elderly get up to pass urine every night, and about half of them need to get up twice. These awakenings, according to the *British Medical Journal* (287:1665), are due to the discomfort of a full bladder and not to insomnia. Insomnia, however often results.

Extra drinking is not responsible, the Journal reports, since elderly people with the same intake as younger people produce relatively more urine at night. Further studies to determine why all elderly people are not similarly affected, and why 30 percent are not troubled at all, would be most important. Could this variation be due to differences in physical activity?

Salt and Insomnia

A common and very easily overlooked cause of insomnia, according to the *Physician and Sports Medicine* (10#9:75). may be an excess of sodium chloride (common salt).

The food eaten by most people in the U.S.A. contains about seven to 15 times more salt than is needed. Without realizing, therefore, we may keep ourselves awake by eating salty food. Since excess sodium is also bad for the blood pressure and heart, here is another reason for cutting down on salt.

Alcohol and Sleep

Not wishing to be dependent on pills, many people who have difficulty sleeping take a drink of liquor, beer, or wine before going to bed, a remedy that, *Geriatrics* (41#6:81) reports, can be counterproductive.

While alcohol is definitely a sedative and can be counted upon to make one quickly fall asleep, this effect can wear off after just a few hours and be replaced by a phase of stimulation and irritability that keeps one awake. It is also true that while small to moderate amounts of alcohol are sedative in effect and make one feel drowsy, larger amounts taken over a prolonged period can, in some cases, actually interfere with sleep.

Alcohol at bedtime may also increase the effect of other medications, such as those that lower blood pressure, antihistamines, heart medicines that relax the arteries, sedatives and tranquilizers The combined effect may produce dizziness and falls, with the risk of a fractured hip or other broken bones, when the person gets out of bed during the night. Alcohol as a sleep aid, therefore, is not a very good idea.

Self Help for Night Cramps

Within seven days, a simple exercise, according to a report in the *New England Journal of Medicine*, cured all of 44 patients who complained of severe night cramping in the legs.

Facing a wall and standing in bare feet with the arms stretched sideways at shoulder level, you slowly lean forwards until you feel a tight pulling sensation in the calf muscles Carried out for a few minutes three times every day, this exercise is a very reasonable first-line treatment for night cramps. If, despite it, cramps persist, then ask for medical help.

Jet Lag Explained

After flying east or west over several time zones, most people do not overcome the "jet lag" for several days. Out of step with their environment, they feel the urge to eat and sleep on the schedule they followed at home. Since traveling the same distance north and south involves no time zone change, there is no jet lag.

This is not only because of a difference in the person's sleeping pattern, but also because it changes the time of day when the hormones in the body, such as adrenalin and thyroid, are most plentiful. Hormone production cannot change suddenly and can only adjust by about one hour a day, as we pointed out in the article "Shift Work and Hormones" under the heading Hormones. Since hormone blood levels can't peak in synchrony with the changed hours of the traveler, the person experiences jet lag.

Surprisingly, more time is needed to overcome jet lag after an eastward journey than after an equally long journey westward. This "directional asymmetry," according to the *British Medical Journal* (284:144), is due to the fact that traveling westwards results in a longer day than usual during the journey, whereas traveling eastwards shortens the day. The human body, research has shown, prefers a long day to a short one. People living without clocks and in a building without windows naturally adopt a sleep-wake cycle of 25 hours or longer in preference to the 24-hour day.

INTESTINAL GAS

Solutions for Intestinal Gas

Those who worry about passing flatus (rectal gas) must understand that it is quite normal to do so, *Drug Therapy* (17#10:76) reports. Everyone experiences this problem to a certain extent, and the amount of gas is excessive only when it causes physical discomfort or bloating of the abdomen.

Gas is produced in the colon (large intestine) by bacteria that ferment the sugars and other carbohydrates which fail to get digested and absorbed higher up in the intestinal tract. One of the more common causes of this embarrassing problem is lactase insufficiency (milk intolerance), a condition in which certain people are incapable of digesting lactose (the natural sugar in milk) because they lack the necessary sugar-splitting enzyme, lactase.

Lactase insufficiency victims can now take the missing enzyme by mouth in the form of the product Lactaid. This is available in drug stores and does not require a prescription.

Other common causes for fermentable sugar reaching the colon include the consumption of wheat, oats, potatoes, or corn in excessive amounts. Some fruits (apricots, bananas, prunes, and raisins) and vegetables (beans, Brussels sprouts, carrots, celery, and onions), contain indigestible carbohydrates, too, and are notorious sources of excessive gas.

However, people differ enormously in how much of these foods they can eat without experiencing this problem. Furthermore, everyone changes in this regard from day to day, and these differences depend upon variation in the types and number of bacteria living in the colon. For those who continue to be plagued by too much gas despite dietary adjustment, one can attempt to reduce the number of the offending colonic bacteria with a short course of antibiotic treatment (a doctor's prescription is needed for this).

First, though, it is worth trying to inhibit the excessive fermentation by taking some charcoal pills by mouth. Activated charcoal (available in most drug stores) is not only a good poison antidote but reduces the bloating and cramps due to excessive intestinal gas, the *American Journal of Gastroenterology* (81:532) reports. In both settings, charcoal works because it absorbs and inactivates many other substances, including gases. This is much less expensive and does not require a doctor's prescription.

By taking some charcoal every day, which is not expensive and does not require a doctor's prescription, one can soon rid oneself of the discomfort and embarrassment of intestinal gas.

KIDNEY PROBLEMS

Aspirin and the Kidneys

Aspirin is one of the non-steroidal anti-inflammatory drugs (NSAIDs), a group of medications used in the symptomatic treatment of arthritis and many other causes of mild to moderate pain. Other drugs included in this group are Indomethacin, Motrin, Nalfon, Naprosyn, and Tolectin. Since they are "non-steroidal" (not like cortisone), they lack many of the undesirable properties of cortisone-like drugs, such as cortisone's ability to raise the blood pressure, weaken the bones, depress immunity, and to mask infections

The NSAIDs, however, have some serious side effects of their own, and one of these is a type of kidney damage, which occurs in about 1 percent of people treated with these drugs, particularly if they are taken for a long time. For this reason, some people are afraid to take an aspirin every day to slow blood clotting and hence to help reduce their risks of coronary heart attack and stroke.

That worry, according to correspondence in the *Lancet* (1:736), is an unnecessary one, since aspirin differs from all the other NSAIDs in that it lacks any ability to harm the kidneys when taken in usual doses by mouth. The reason for this is that aspirin is broken down by digestion in the intestine and further changed in the liver immediately after absorption so that, after usual dosages by mouth, not enough intact aspirin gets into the general circulation to harm the kidneys.

Dialysis or Kidney Transplant?

When kidney failure progresses to the point where urinary waste products accumulate in the bloodstream, either dialysis or a kidney transplant is required. At different times, both may be needed by the same patient. During the first year, for instance, rather than accepting the first available kidney, which may not match well with the recipient's tissues, it may be safer to continue dialysis until a kidney which matches well becomes available.

However, the record of the hospital where dialysis is being given should be taken into account. For instance, according to *Medical World News* (22#25:16), the success of dialysis (as measured by the percentage of patients surviving one year), varies from hospital to hospital by as much as from 55 to 85 percent.

After the first year, the success of dialysis falls so dramatically that a transplant then offers a much better chance of survival, even with a kidney that does not closely match the host's tissues. Three-year transplant survival can vary between 65 and 85 percent, depending on how well the tissues match.

Worcestershire Sauce and Kidney Damage

Both adults and children can seriously harm their kidneys with Worcestershire sauce if they sprinkle it on their meat regularly and too liberally. *American Family Physician* (27#2:347) recently quoted other medical journals on this topic and pointed out that the symptoms and signs (including blood in the urine) that are caused by excessive use of this sauce indicate quite serious damage to the kidneys. Eventually, this clears up if use of the sauce is discontinued. To be safe, therefore, use it very sparingly.

MONONUCLEOSIS

Persisting Mononucleosis

Forty-four people (adults and children) who have remained unwell for as long as one year were recently described in the *Annals of Internal Medicine* (102:1&7). Their symptoms have included sore throat, fever, swollen and tender lymph nodes in the neck and elsewhere, aching joints, slow thinking, tiredness, physical fatigue, and a feeling of gloom. They were generally unwell without first having gone through any recognizable acute illness.

Investigation of these people with blood tests revealed the presence in their tissues of the Epstein-Barr (EB) virus, which, among other things, is responsible for mononucleosis. The illness from which they were suffering is known as the chronic mononucleosis syndrome (CMS).

Mononucleosis of such gradual onset and persistence is not usual. Why, in such cases, the body cannot rid itself of the EB virus is not understood. To date, there is no treatment for CMS, but extra rest seems to help us cope better with its symptoms. After several months to a year, most of the patients begin to feel better, but in a few cases, the illness lasts even longer.

The behavior of children with vague fatigue, and who seem to have lost all interest in school, has often been attributed to some emotional difficulty. Now, *Pediatric Notes* (9:24) suggests, one of the first things to think about is testing them for CMS.

MOUTH PROBLEMS

Tea Bags for Bleeding in the Mouth

The bleeding from an injured tongue, even when it merely results from an accidental self-inflected bite, is often prolonged and alarming. Usually though, such bleeding can quickly be brought under control, without stitches or help from a doctor, if the victim firmly holds something over the site of bleeding to compress it. A wet handkerchief or face towel is commonly used for this purpose at home, while sterile gauze tends to be used in hospitals. Either type of packing material will be satisfactory if compression is sufficient and is kept up for a long enough time.

Now, however, *Emergency Medicine* (18#18:16) reports, quicker control over the bleeding can be achieved if one presses a wet tea bag against the wound. The tannin of the tea leaves, apparently, has a coagulating property that promotes more rapid clotting of the blood. With advantage, one can still put a handkerchief, etc., over the tea bag to make sure that sufficient pressure is brought to bear upon the bleeding laceration.

Bad Breath

While it is true that disease in almost any part of the body can cause bad breath (halitosis), over 90 percent of cases stem from local conditions in the mouths of otherwise normal people, the Finnish medical journal, *Suomen Laakarilehti* (40:2309) reports. Most of the remainder have an abnormal lung condition, and only very few have a "general" illness that taints both the bloodstream and breath, such as liver or kidney failure, or diabetes.

To determine whether bad breath is coming from the mouth or from elsewhere, exhale deeply through the nostrils with the mouth shut. If another person can detect an odor on the breath under these conditions, it must be coming from the lungs, the *U.S. Pharmacist* (10#10:24) reports.

Conversely, bad breath detectable when one exhales gently through the mouth with the nostrils closed must be coming from the mouth. Mouth conditions giving rise to halitosis include poor hygiene with putrefying food particles between the teeth, dental caries or plaque, and inflammation of the gums or gum pockets that harbor rotting food. Bad breath from these causes, of course, can usually be dealt with by dentists.

Another mouth condition frequently overlooked as a cause of bad breath is the growth of fungus or yeast over the top of the tongue, making it appear coated or "hairy," a problem that can usually be eliminated by brushing the tongue when one is cleaning the teeth.

Older people who take good care of their mouths may

nevertheless have bad breath, the *Journal of the American Medical Association* (254:2473) reports, since they do not produce sufficient saliva. The resulting oral dryness allows odor-producing bacteria to flourish between their teeth. The remedy for this problem is to use a mouthwash or an artificial saliva spray between meals.

Lastly, dryness of the air inside a house may be making a contribution to bad breath since it leads to crusting of mucus and excessive bacterial growth in the nose and mouth, especially in elderly people, who already have some nasal and oral dryness. Dryness of the air, however, can easily be eliminated with a humidifier. *Consumer Reports* (50:679) recommends the ultrasonic type of humidifier since, unlike the others, it spreads very few bacteria.

Mouth Dryness

Aging, Sjogren's Disease (an illness involving dry mouth, dry eyes, and painful joints), certain medications, and radiation treatment over the salivary glands — all result in excessive dryness of the mouth. The mouth-drying effect of certain medicines, understandably, is temporary, but dryness of the mouth due to all of the other causes listed above is permanent. Dryness of the mouth is medically known as xerostomia.

Ordinarily just a nuisance, dryness of the mouth can become dangerous if one has angina pectoris (pain in the chest due to heart disease) and relies upon a tablet of nitroglycerin put under the tongue, where it should quickly dissolve and be absorbed for relief. Also, according to *Geriatrics* (38#5:16), dryness of the mouth can result in tooth decay if left untreated.

The remedy, of course, is to moisten the mouth by

drinking frequently or, better still, by using one of the salivary substitute products, such as Salivart or Xero-Lube, which provide not only water but also certain elements normally present in saliva. Salivary substitute spray products that can be carried in the pocket or in the handbag are now available in most drug stores without prescription.

Now, a correspondent to the *New England Journal of Medicine* (310:1122) suggests, relief from drug-induced mouth dryness can be even more easily obtained by swallowing tablets of another medication called Bethanechol, which stimulates the salivary flow. A doctor's prescription is needed for these pills.

Tonsils and Interferon

Traditionally, the tonsils have been thought of as vestigial organs that, like the appendix, are useless to modern man. Now, according to *American Family Physician* (24:244), tonsil tissue turns out to be one of the body's most efficient interferon-producing sites. Part of our immune mechanism, interferon is tailor-made by the body to combat each virus infection as it occurs, thereby helping to stamp it out and limit its duration.

Since people who have had their tonsils out can still cope well with infections, other tissues of the body must be able to take over this function.

NOISE SENSITIVITY

Noise and Behavior

How does noise affect our behavior? One interesting fact, according to the *British Medical Journal* (281:1325), is that brown eyed people are less affected by noise than are those with blue eyes. There is not a clear explanation why this is so.

The article also points out the difference background noise can make in our perception of a loud noise. In one experiment someone dropped a pile of books on a busy sidewalk, both in quiet surroundings and in noisy ones. When done in quiet surroundings, 20 percent of passers-by helped pick them up, but in the presence of intense noise only 10 percent helped. When the book dropper wore a plaster cast, the difference was amplified, with 80 percent of passers-by helping when it was quiet, but only 15 percent when it was noisy.

Coping with noise, it seems, blunts our ability to perceive.

ORAL CONTRACEPTIVES

Failure of Oral Contraceptives

Women who use "the Pill" should be aware that other medicines can counteract the effect of oral contraceptives. Certain anti-arthritis drugs and pain relievers, sedatives, anti-convulsants, and sleeping pills commonly do this.

Anti-infectives (sulfa drugs and antibiotics) are the most widely used medications to have this effect, *Modern Medicine* (55#5:189) reports. Women who take Bactrim or Septra for bladder or kidney infections, for example, are more likely to become pregnant while on such medication and should employ an additional contraceptive method (such as abstinence or a diaphragm) for so long as they continue to take the anti-infective drug. Medications reduce an oral contraceptive's efficiency either by interfering with its absorption or by increasing its rate of destruction by the liver.

Accordingly, if one is taking "the Pill," and the doctor orders additional medication, ask him about this possible interaction.

Deafness and the Pill

It has long been known that pregnancy can hasten the onset of deafness in members of certain families who have a tendency to gradual hearing loss in middle age. Known as otosclerosis, this common type of deafness is due to overgrowth of bone around the inner eardrum, which becomes rigid and unable to vibrate in response to sound.

Nowadays, otosclerosis is cured by the operation called fenestration, in which a new inner eardrum is artificially created. The latest news on this front is that oral contraceptive (OC) drugs can bring on otosclerosis. Since OCs highly resemble natural hormones that are produced during pregnancy, this is not surprising.

For this reason, the *British Journal of Family Planning* (9:134) suggests that, before starting on an OC, women should have hearing tests and be asked if there is deafness in the family. Those with any tendency to otosclerosis or with a family history of deafness should avoid OCs entirely.

OSTEOPOROSIS

Osteoporosis — A Serious Disease

Osteoporosis is the medical term for a weakening of the bones which often occurs with aging. It is responsible for many hip and arm fractures and collapse of the vertebrae (spinal bones), with gradual loss of height and curvature of the back ("dowager's hump").

Such skeletal softening has been attributed mostly to loss of calcium and phosphorus from the body. However, as we shall see in the following articles, other factors play a part as well.

The incidence of osteoporosis rises most dramatically in women after the menopause. For this reason the disease has been linked with hormonal changes, and many women take estrogen to prevent osteoporosis. Others fear that this may bring on cancer of the uterus, so they hesitate to take the hormones. For more information about this very important question, please read the article, "Should Women Take Estrogens to Prevent Osteoporosis?" in the section of the book on Hormones.

Antacids and Osteoporosis

Aluminum-containing antacids, if used regularly, tend to cause extensive loss of calcium and phosphorus from the body, thereby seriously weakening the bones. X-rays of a 60-year-old woman with limb pains and excessive weakness revealed that her bones had lost so much density that they were scarcely able to support her tissues. Her osteoporosis, according to the *Journal of the American Medical Association* (244:2544), was due to the long-term daily use of an antacid containing aluminum hydroxide.

Antacids that contain aluminum, *Archives of Internal Medicine* (143:657) reports, can become a major factor in weakening the bones. However, since they do not produce any noticeable unpleasant side effects, people continue taking them for stomach pains and indigestion.

These drugs work by binding and neutralizing gastric acid. Unfortunately, they also bind with and prevent the absorption of phosphoric acid, which is then carried away in the stools. To compensate the body for this, the bones release some phosphorus into the bloodstream, together with the calcium with which it was bound. This calcium is quickly carried away through the kidneys.

In this way, aluminum antacids taken year after year can deplete the skeleton of calcium and phosphorus and cause thinning and weakness of all the bones. This results in fractures occurring in response to only trivial trauma, and to pseudofractures, a condition in which bones crack but do not break completely, causing weakness, pain, and stiffness that are often mistaken for arthritis.

Doctors, more and more, are becoming aware of this danger, but aluminum-containing antacids are still widely prescribed and can be purchased without prescription. The trouble is that it takes years for the cumulative bad effects of repeated doses to show up and, later in life, people tend to accept bone pain and fractures as a natural effect of aging.

To compensate for this danger, the *Archives* recommends, we should take extra calcium and phosphorus when using medications that contain aluminum or, better still, take stom ach medicines that are aluminum-free. Aluminum, remember, poses other serious threats as well (see, for example, the articles on Alzheimer's Disease). One of the least expensive and most readily available forms of calcium in tablet form is the antacid Tums. Before purchasing an antacid, read the list of ingredients on the labeling. The pharmacist can tell you about products that are aluminum-free.

Smoking and Osteoporosis

Smoking, a Mayo Clinic expert on bone disease reports in the *New England Journal of Medicine* (314:181), makes osteoporosis much more pronounced and accounts for a greater than two-fold increase in hip and arm fractures and vertebral collapse.

Until now, osteoporosis has been considered to be essentially a disease of elderly women. According to the expert quoted above, however, older men, too, can suffer from quite pronounced osteoporosis, especially if they smoke.

Calcium and Osteoporosis

Nowadays, with so much emphasis being put on the need to reduce the fat in our food and to increase our dietary intake of fiber and bulk-producing vegetables, care must be taken to avoid a deficiency of calcium.

Fat-containing dairy products, especially milk and ice cream, used to provide us with most of our calcium, whereas the vegetables and cereals, which we are now taking in their place, bind with calcium in the intestines and thus interfere with its absorption, *Medical World News* (25#12:41) reports. The net result, if we are not careful, is a calcium deficiency that leaves our bones weaker and more brittle than usual and unusually prone to be fractured, even in response to minor trauma.

While no one denies that low fat and high fiber diets benefit us by greatly reducing our liability to heart disease and stroke, we must take care to compensate for the decreased availability of calcium they bring about. We can help ourselves by taking, in addition to our one vitamin-mineral pill a day, half a gram (500 mg) tablet of calcium carbonate three times daily (or four times if one is big) as well.

It is important to note that it matters when we take these tablets. Since the calcium in pills can only be absorbed if there is a normal amount of acid in the stomach, the *Journal of the American Medical Association* (257:541) reports that older people, whose stomachs no longer produce much acid, cannot benefit from taking calcium between meals. Taken with food, however, calcium is absorbed, regardless of the lack of gastric acid.

Another article in the *Journal of the American Medical Association* (247:1106) emphasizes that taking calcium alone is not enough and, even in optimal amounts, can do nothing to prevent the bones from becoming osteoporotic in people who are inactive. Both exercise and calcium are needed to restore osteoporotic bones. Because exercise (e.g., walking two miles every day) can be difficult or impossible for those who have already become disabled by osteoporosis, prevention is truly better than cure.

Also, according to the *Mayo Clinic Proceedings* (61:116), it has been discovered that the density and amount of calcium in an older woman's spinal bones correlates very closely with the strength of her back muscles. Thus, it is believed, older women may be able to protect themselves against collapse of the spinal bones by regularly performing exercises that increase the tone of the back muscles. Although it will take many years to obtain final proof that this works, it is reasonable for women to perform daily back exercises (sit-ups or with a rowing machine), so long as they do not overexert or hurt themselves.

Manganese and Osteoporosis

Manganese is perhaps no less important than calcium for maintaining the strength of the bones, according to *Science News* (130:199). In fact, that journal reports, the only abnormality consistently found in the blood of a group of women with osteoporosis was an extremely low level of manganese.

Furthermore, a young basketball superstar who was constantly plagued with stress fractures and found to have osteoporosis was also found to have a low level of manganese. This was attributed to a special diet that he was taking. His blood calcium level, incidentally, was normal. After he was put on a dietary supplement of minerals to correct his blood levels of manganese and some other elements, his bones healed, and he had no more fractures.

Health food stores nowadays stock tablets containing five mg of manganese (or 50 mg of manganese gluconate, which is equivalent), enough to prevent manganese deficiency (and presumably osteoporosis) if taken every day, *Science News* reports. If one is also taking a supplement of calcium, take manganese at a different time of day, since these substances compete with one another for absorption.

Anorexia Nervosa and Osteoporosis

Anorexia nervosa, the illness in which young women who have been dieting strenuously become abnormally thin and unable to regain weight, often also causes profound calcium loss from the bones. This loss, which is noticeable in X-rays, often reveals that the victims have osteoporosis.

Interestingly, it was found that osteoporosis develops only in those anorexia nervosa patients who become inactive or who spend most of their time in bed. Others, who stay up and about and remain very active, have little bone thinning and no fractures. Physical inactivity, then, has much to do with the patient's recovery, and bed rest, a treatment often prescribed for these women until now is to be no longer recommended.

Another cause of osteoporosis in these patients, according to the *New England Journal of Medicine* (311:1601), is a reduction in the amount of estrogen (feminizing hormone) produced by the emaciated women, because during the strenuous dieting their periods stop also. The *Journal* reports that by giving estrogen to restore their natural tissue levels of this hormone, one may help them to conserve calcium and the strength of their bones.

For more information on this disease, see the section on Anorexia Nervosa.

PAIN

Imagined Pain Relief Is Real

About one in three persons can obtain pain relief with sugar pills. This so-called "placebo effect" (pla-see'bo, which in Latin means, "I shall please") works only if the patients believe that they are getting real medication.

Even so, this is no laughing matter, particularly now that we understand how placebos work. University of California researchers report in *Lancet* that placebo pain relief can be wiped out by injecting naloxone, a drug that is normally used as an antidote for narcotic overdosage.

This strongly suggests that the brain of a placebo-responder makes its own narcotic-like substance, and it is this that relieves pain when a placebo is given. Testing this theory further, the researchers took people whose pain normally responded to placebo and pretreated them with naloxone. No pain relief could then be obtained with placebo.

After repeated use over long periods, placebos become less effective and patients with persisting pain need ever larger numbers of sugar pills each succeeding day. This growing "tolerance" is seen also with narcotics.

Menthol Ointments and Heating Pads

Menthol-containing ointment (such as Ben-Gay or Vicks) that is rubbed on skin to relieve muscular or arthritic pain must never be used with a heating pad, the manufacturers warn.

Modern Medicine (55#10:137) tells the sad story of a man who disregarded this advice and ended up in a hospital for one year. After applying the ointment to his aching thighs and forearms, he held a heating pad over each treated area for 15-20 minutes.

Next day, the treated skin appeared inflamed and was covered with large blisters, a reaction that did not respond to cortisone. Over the next few days he became feverish and lost all of the skin, fat, and underlying connective tissues down to the muscles (which became fully exposed) at all of the treated sites. His kidneys were permanently injured, too. During his year-long hospital stay, he needed repeated surgery to clean the "burned" sites and repair them with full thickness skin grafts.

The moral of this story: Read the labeling of all medicines and follow the instructions carefully.

Music Practice

When musicians suddenly increase the duration and intensity of practice or playing they risk getting the overuse syndrome, a disorder that causes pain, weakness, and loss of function in certain muscles, the *Lancet* (2:728) reports. Playing string instruments causes this problem to occur in the upper limbs, but, with wind instruments, it is the lips, tongue, throat, and chest that are affected. In severe cases, stiffening and deformity may occur, with arthritis in the joints of the hands, arm, or spine.

To avoid the problem, musicians should not play continuously for long periods. Parents and teachers of children learning to play an instrument should not insist upon unbroken hour-long sessions of practice. Sporting activity and exercises that extend the range of motion of the spine and strengthen the muscles are helpful. Any repertoire that brings on pain or discomfort should be abandoned.

Lastly, supporting devices that take the weight of an instrument off the musicians' arms can make a considerable difference. If partial resting fails to alleviate the pain and tenderness, the musician should give up playing completely for many months, until all of the symptoms have disappeared altogether. Other activities (e.g: writing or turning taps) that also bring on the symptoms must be abandoned, too. Medical care is necessary.

Only after the symptoms have cleared completely can the musician safely resume playing, starting with one minute twice daily and extending the time very gradually. Since the overuse syndrome can be so disabling and difficult to overcome, music performers need to be alert to the danger of playing for too long.

PREMENSTRUAL TENSION SYNDROME (PMS)

Coffee and PMS

Confirmation of the link between coffee drinking and PMS comes from a study published in the *American Journal of Public Health* (75#11:1335). Drinking coffee aggravates the symptoms to such an extent that a woman for whom PMS is a problem should be very careful about her intake, especially just before the onset of her period.

The symptoms of this troublesome but not dangerous condition include tiredness, irritability, anxiety, depression, headaches, tender and swollen breasts, constipation, acne, and a craving for salty or sweet food. Many women also have backache, swelling of the abdomen, fingers and ankles, and a decreased tolerance for alcohol.

One or more of these symptoms occur with every menstrual cycle for a few days before the flow and then cease. Though more study is needed, and coffee is certainly not the only offender, women who are bothered by PMS to could try to reduce their coffee drinking during this time of the month.

POISONING

Lead Poisoning

Until some time early in this century, pewter was made by mixing tin with lead, the *British Medical Journal* (291:1701) reports. Although the risk of lead poisoning from old pewter dishes is minimal, pewter tankards, mugs, or cups are much more dangerous because, if used repeatedly, their fluid contents dissolve a lot of lead. Since modern pewter vessels contain no lead, they can be used without risk.

Nonetheless, the *Western Journal of Medicine* (143:357) reports, modern pottery colored with lead-containing pigments may not be safe, even if the covering glaze appears to be intact, since it often becomes scratched off or cracked. Furthermore, even some glazes contain lead. People who color pottery or paint with lead-containing pigments (such as cinnabar) are also at risk and must wash their hands before touching their mouths or handling food.

Symptoms of lead poisoning from such sources include mood changes, headache, aching of the limbs, constipation, and bouts of colicky abdominal pain. Since lead poisoning is quite common, anyone having these symptoms should ask a doctor to check them over with this cause in mind.

Castor Oil Beans Cause Death

Not long ago, a Bulgarian political refugee in London died three days after a mysterious stranger jabbed him in the leg with a sharpened umbrella tip. Autopsy revealed a minute hollow pellet deep in his wound that, it was believed, contained a fatal poison.

From the nature of his slow death, it was determined that this substance was ricin, an intensely toxic substance (more poisonous than snake venom) present in the castor oil bean. It is not present in castor oil but remains in the bean "cake" after the oil has been extracted. The cake can be rendered safe for human consumption by cooking and is used as staple food in several parts of the world, including Mexico.

Mexicans and Caribbean islanders employ the attractive looking castor oil bean to make necklaces and other jewelry for the tourist trade. According to Toxicology, there have been serious reactions and deaths when people have eaten one of these beans or have merely crushed one in their fingers and subsequently put their fingers in their mouths. Ricin causes drastic purging with bloody diarrhea, shivering, fever, violent vomiting, and shock. Even a minute trace in a scratch can be fatal. So, when shopping abroad for trinkets, avoid buying castor oil bean jewelry.

Toad Poisoning

While petting frogs is a harmless childhood activity, handling toads can be dangerous, the *New England Journal of Medicine* (314:1517) reports, since the skin of some types of toad secretes a poison which, when conveyed to the mouth, causes drooling, convulsive seizures, and serious disturbances of the heart rhythm. The Colorado River toad is the most toxic toad in North America and well-known as the cause of neurological problems and even death in animals that pick it up by mouth.

Now, according to the *Journal*, a young boy who played with a toad of this type required intensive care in a hospital for over seven days before he began to recover from paralysis, seizures, and difficulty in breathing, and probably would have died without such treatment.

Accordingly, while it is quite safe for children to play with frogs, don't let them ever even touch a toad. Telling frogs and toads apart, however, may not always be so easy.

Wild Plant Poisoning

As more and more people take up wilderness river rafting as a means of getting back to nature, the number of plant poisoning cases has been on the increase. Ingestion of the water hemlock plant (known as Cicuta douglasii), the *Western Journal of Medicine* (142:637) reports, has recently been responsible for the deaths of several river rafters in Oregon and Idaho.

This plant closely resembles the wild carrot or parsnip. It has large fleshy roots with a smell so strongly suggestive of carrots and celery that people are tempted to taste them.

Unfortunately, however, the water hemlock is one of our most poisonous wild plants and can bring on convulsions, collapse, and death, all within an hour or two after one has taken a small bite of its root.

About the only method of treating hemlock poisoning available in the wilderness is the induction of vomiting, but, without an emetic such as syrup of ipecac, this can be very difficult. Campers, therefore, should always be prepared for such emergencies by carrying a reliable emetic in their packs.

In emergencies, a useful trick that can save lives from poisoning, according to the *Journal*, is to make up an emetic by mixing a tablespoonful of liquid dish soap in eight ounces of water.

Potato Poisoning

Thanks to their bitter taste, potato stems and leaves are rarely eaten. This is fortunate because all parts of a potato plant except its root tubers (the potatoes) contain the potent poison, solanine. High concentrations of solanine are produced in the shoots of potatoes; and the potatoes themselves, as well as their shoots, become loaded with solanine a few days after they begin sprouting.

Vomiting and diarrhea, sometimes accompanied by mild fever, appear four to 14 hours after ingestion of sprouting potatoes. Large amounts of solanine can cause coma, convulsions and circulatory collapse, from which some people never recover. According to the *Quarterly Journal of Medicine*, the diarrhea and vomiting last for about a week, while mental confusion and hallucinations may persist for several more days after physical recovery. People already weakened by heart disease, alcoholism, or malnutrition, etc., are the most likely to be fatally affected.

Two points worth making are that mild solanine poisoning may be the unrecognized cause of institutional diarrhea outbreaks and that no amount of cooking can remove solanine from potatoes once it has been formed. So, be on the safe side, and throw away any potatoes that are beginning to sprout.

Salad Dressing for Picnic Safety

Knowledge of some of the basic facts about food perishability can help one avoid food poisoning on picnics, *Indiana Medicine* (79:360) reports. Because the bacteria that cause food poisoning cannot flourish or even survive for long in acid surroundings, special precautions are necessary with foods that are low in acid, such as chicken, ham, eggs, and potatoes, all of which are common ingredients for sandwiches and summer meals outdoors. As most readers already know, these foods should be taken out of the refrigerator at the last moment and kept in an insulated cooler next to a frozen ice can.

It is not so well known, however, that mayonnaise and salad dressing, by virtue of their lemon juice and vinegar ingredients, are strongly acidic and therefore help prevent the growth of bacteria that cause food poisoning. Thus, the sooner that mayonnaise or salad dressing can be added to non-acid foods and salad materials after they are taken from the refrigerator, the lesser is the chance that food will be spoiled by dangerous bacteria.

Fish Poisoning

Common in Florida from early February through late August every year, outbreaks of ciguatera fish poisoning occur after ingestion of certain types of ocean fish, especially grouper and snapper. Beginning two to 30 hours after a meal, this illness usually starts with diarrhea and vomiting, which may cause such severe dehydration that hospitalization for intravenous fluid treatment becomes necessary. Some victims first complain of itching, with weakness and aching of the legs and thighs. Sooner or later, nearly everyone experiences reversal of temperature sensations (cold fluids in the mouth feel hot), hypersensitivity of the teeth, and sensations of burning in the palms and soles. Although many ciguatera fish poisoning victims may continue to feel weak for many months, fatalities have not been reported.

The larger and more mature fish, according to the *Journal of the American Medical Association* (244:254) are more likely to cause ciguatera poisoning. For this reason, Floridians have learned to avoid big specimens of grouper and snapper during the season of risk. Since frozen fish can be stored for many months and is trucked all over the country, avoid grouper or snapper unless you are in Florida and can be certain that it has been freshly caught during safe months of the year.

Poisoning by Household Insecticides

During the past 20 years, American apple-growers and farmers have more than doubled their use of insecticides containing organophosphates, carbamates, propoxur or pyrethins, and, at the same time, have suffered increasingly from aplastic anemia and leukemia.

Although there is no proof of cause-and-effect, according to a *Lancet* (2:300) report, the evidence strongly suggests that many of these potentially fatal bone marrow disorders result from exposure to insecticide mist or fog. Malathion, DDVP,

Raid, Holiday Fogger, and Baygon were among the household insecticides to which the aplastic anemia and leukemia victims were exposed.

Children, it seems, are much more susceptible than adults, and insecticide inhalation is more dangerous for them than is contact with the skin. Most victims were exposed to mist or fog for only a few hours and did not begin to feel unwell until several days or weeks later.

Mothballs

Napthalene not only repels moths but it also helps to keep away most other insects. Its strong smell, too, can mask odors. For these reasons, according to *Morbidity and Mortality Reports* (32:34), mothballs are commonly used indoors in some parts of the country to control odors and insects.

This practice is unsafe and should be stopped because napthalene particles are absorbed into the body through the lungs and skin and have very toxic effects. Included among these are skin and eye irritation, nausea, vomiting, abdominal cramps, diarrhea and, depending upon the concentration, anemia, excitement, confusion, convulsions, jaundice, and kidney failure.

PSORIASIS

The Good Side of Psoriasis

Although the unsightly scaling red skin of psoriasis impairs self-image and is often accompanied by arthritis, it is now thought to be a sign of immunity against skin cancer and probably against cancer in other parts of the body too.

Despite repeated treatments with ultraviolet light and tar-containing ointments, both of which are known carcinogens (cancer producers), the skin of psoriatic patients, according to the *International Journal of Cancer*, rarely becomes cancerous.

Furthermore, it has been noted, among white Australian farmers who spend most of their time outdoors in the sunshine, the incidence of solar keratosis (a skin cancer precursor) is only 4 percent in those who have psoriasis as against 88 percent of those with normal skin.

Hepatitis and Psoriasis

Hepatitis B, the type of viral hepatitis that is conveyed from person to person in "biological fluids," is a potential risk of transfusions when the blood obtained from an unknown donor who might be a hepatitis carrier.

Normally, we would not expect to become infected with this virus merely by touching surfaces that have been contaminated with fluid droplets from a carrier, unless our skin at the contact site had been scratched, cut, or pricked (thereby simulating the conditions of a transfusion or injection). Now, however, the *British Medical Journal* (284:84) points out, the skin of eczema or psoriasis victims is so permeable that, even without injury, it allows virus particles to pass through into the body's interior. To avoid such infection, therefore, the *Journal* article recommends that chronic skin disease victims should be immunized with the new Hepatitis B vaccine.

Since many other potentially dangerous microorganisms

lurk in moisture droplets on all kinds of surfaces, particularly in public places, people with chronic skin diseases should make a habit of touching things away from home as little as possible and should carefully wash and dry the skin whenever such contact is unavoidable.

SKIN PROBLEMS

Vitiligo

About 1-2 percent of the population exhibits a failure of pigmentation in patches of the skin which, as a consequence, appear unnaturally white. While in a few cases, the lack of pigmentation is generalized, the white patches are usually only a few inches across and occur on the parts of the body that are most exposed. The face (especially around the mouth and eyes), neck, chest, armpits, elbows, and knees are most affected.

Treatment, which, the *American Family Physician* (33#5:137) reports, is often unsatisfactory, includes repeated exposure to ultraviolet light after the patient has been given psoralen, a drug that sensitizes skin and makes it more reactive to sunlight. Before this, however, the eyes must be examined by an expert since the retina may also be involved in this pigment disturbance and could be injured by the psoralen-light reaction. Some parts of the skin may pigment more deeply and permanently than others in response to treatment. Skin that does not darken can be hidden with cosmetics or, alternatively, the surrounding skin can be lightened with

Eldoquin or Artra creams to blur the edges of the patches and make them less noticeable.

It is essential that anyone with patches of de pigmented skin be seen by a dermatologist, since there are other conditions, including some types of poisoning and serious infection, that resemble vitiligo but that urgently need very different treatment. Moreover, anyone with vitiligo should undergo very careful medical examination, because in some cases there is an associated major illness, such as an autoimmunity (in which the tissues attack themselves), diabetes, thyroid disease, pernicious anemia, myasthenia gravis, or melanoma. The relationship with melanoma is intriguing since a melanoma is a cancer of pigment-producing skin cells. However, having vitiligo does not mean that one is likely to develop a melanoma; the reverse is true and about 20 percent of melanoma patients also have vitiligo. Furthermore, the occurrence of vitiligo in someone who has had a melanoma removed sometimes heralds the development of recurrent melanoma tumors elsewhere in the body (i.e: in the liver).

Creeping Eruption

Creeping eruption is the intensely itching skin disease caused by tiny parasitic worms (the larvae of insects) crawling around just under the surface of the skin. Wandering aimlessly, the larvae move about one inch daily, leaving irregular, red, slightly raised tracks in the skin rather like miniature mole tunnels.

Also known as Cutaneous Larva Migrans, this condition occurs when human skin is parasitized by the eggs of worms that normally infest other species (e.g: dog, cat, or cattle hookworms), the *American Family Physician* (35#6:163) reports. The same sort of situation arises when horse flies or deer flies lay eggs in human skin, but the resulting maggots that hatch and live there are much larger and cause "hot spot" lesions that resemble boils.

Larvae remain trapped under the surface of our skin only if their species are not adapted to ours. When "human" hookworms get into us, however, the larvae not only causes redness and irritation at the site of entry through the skin, but they soon move on through the bloodstream to the lungs (temporarily producing cough and bloody sputum) to settle ultimately in our intestines. There they develop into adult worms that cause us to bleed internally and become anemic. Only when parasites are in the wrong species are they unable to migrate and to complete their life cycles.

Fortunately, when any of these conditions is recognized, it can be cured with appropriate medications. The moral of this story, then, is to visit a dermatologist without delay if creams do not quickly take care of itchy red lesions of the skin.

Wart Removal

Warts are local accumulations of skin cells which have become abnormally large and adherent to one another as the result of infection with one of nine possible wart viruses. In people whose warts have become widespread and unusually persistent (warts normally disappear in about nine months), an additional factor — decreased immunity — is also at work.

Treatment of common warts on the hands and fingers, according to the *Resident and Staff Physician* (26:58), need not be traumatic to be effective. Even applications of relatively mild lotions, such as salicylic acid, may disturb the walls of the wart cells sufficiently to let some wart virus escape into the patient's bloodstream. This boosts production of antibodies against the virus which eventually attack the warts and destroy them.

So, if you have warts on your fingers, it is better to let your own body deal with them. If you rush to have them burned off, your immunity never gets stimulated and they may quickly come back again.

Dry Skin

Troublesome dryness of the skin can occur as the result of daily bathing or showering, especially in older people. The skin, particularly that over the lower legs, feels itchy and appears white, rough, scaly, even cracked, so that it may bleed and become red and infected.

The best way to deal with this common problem, the *U.S. Pharmacist* (13#12:24) advises, is to first soak the skin in warm (not hot) water for about 10 minutes. After this, the skin must be thoroughly dried with a towel and then, and only then, it should be immediately covered with a film of ointment or cream. The soaking gives time for the water to penetrate into the deepest layers of dry skin and the thin layer of ointment or cream then acts as a barrier to prevent the water from evaporating away. However, since water and oil don't mix, the surface must be completely dried before ointment or cream can be properly applied. Without the soaking, a cream or ointment cannot do much good.

Since ointments are more oily than creams, they form a more lasting water-retaining barrier. However, because ointments are stickier and less easily washed off, creams are more popular, especially during the day. With creams, though, one must be prepared to soak the skin more often.

Containing still less oil, or even none at all, lotions, although soothing, are almost useless for treating skin that is already excessively dry. They may provide some help, of course, in preventing normal skin from becoming dried out. Gels, which usually contain some alcohol, may actually dry the skin.

Cutis (37:384) recommends that we add Alpha Keri oil to our bath water. Those who preferred showering to sitting in the tub got the same benefit from Alpha Keri oil by rubbing it on the skin immediately after drying. Other bath oils probably have the same effect.

Poison Ivy

If you are very sensitive to poison ivy, you can get a severe reaction from even the most fleeting contact with the plant. For instance, by merely stroking a dog whose fur was in contact with an ivy plant several hours previously, you can develop a classic irritating rash, *Cutis* (37#6:434) reports.

In severe cases, despite treatment from a doctor with the strongest cortisone-like medications, itching that is troublesome enough to interfere with sleep can last for several days. Tub baths of 15 to 20 minutes and using a special oatmeal derivative (trade-named Aveeno) in the water, can be sufficiently soothing to allow one to return to bed and fall asleep.

Nickel Dermatitis

An itching rash covered in tiny blisters may occur at points of contact with watch bands, ear rings, and costume jewelry, and then spread widely over the surrounding skin in people who have become sensitive to nickel. This is much more likely to occur when there is excessive perspiration, so that the skin is moist at the point of contact with the metal. In some cases, furthermore, the dermatitis becomes so widespread that it is mistaken for scabies.

The latest news about nickel, *Cutis* (35#5:424) reports, is the mysterious appearance of dermatitis on the abdomen just below the umbilicus. Eventually, its cause was found to be contact with nickel buttons on blue jeans. In many cases, the dermatitis had also spread to other parts of the body. More often than not, treatment of this condition involves nothing more than replacing the button, watch band, etc., with an item made of another material. If the rash is severe and widespread, however, a visit to the dermatologist for special medication is required.

Bubble Bath Dermatitis

Chemicals used in bubble bath products may cause dermatitis and may even irritate the tissues of the lower urinary tract sufficiently to cause hematuria (bloody urine). This, according to *Modern Medicine* (50#3:45), is most likely to occur when people soak in the bath for too long.

Cashew Nut Dermatitis

Morbidity and Mortality Weekly Reports (32:129) mentions an outbreak of poison ivy-like dermatitis that recently affected 54 people in a small Pennsylvania town. All of the victims had eaten cashew nut pieces purchased from the same Little League organization. The rash appeared on their hands, arms, trunk, and in their mouths, lasted about seven days, and affected approximately 20 percent of the people who had consumed the nuts.

The cashew nut tree, apparently, is of the same species as poison ivy, poison oak, and poison sumac. For this reason, cashew nut shells contain the same chemical irritant and must be completely removed from the nuts (which should then be boiled) before they are made available for human consumption. To avoid problems, readers are advised to purchase only those brands of cashew nuts that have been processed by well-established companies that you have had experience with in the past.

Carotenemia

Carotene is the natural yellowish-red pigment in carrots and tomatoes that is also present in many other vegetables, such as broccoli and squash, which do not look yellow at all. Excessive intake of these vegetables results in deposition of the pigment throughout the body and yellowish discoloration of the skin. This is particularly noticeable on the palms and soles and on the cheeks beside the nose. Unlike jaundice (which occurs in liver disease), the whites of the eyes are not affected.

Most cases of carotenemia, the *Journal of the American Medical Association* (247:926) reports, occur in women who do not eat red meat and consume large quantities of raw vegetables instead. Some such women gradually stop having periods long before the menopause and may become sterile, an effect thought to be due to carotene's chemical influence on a part of the brain that controls the ovaries.

Otherwise healthy young women with this problem can expect to start having periods again within about four months, the *Journal* reports, if they alter their diets to decrease the blood level of carotene.

Aloe Vera — Fact or Fiction?

Aloe vera, the Mexican healing plant, is the time-honored home remedy for a variety of human ills, but very few doctors know anything about it. For this reason, the journal *Cutis* (37:106) recently reviewed the plant's chemical ingredients and pointed out that many of them are medicinally active. For instance, aloe contains an enzyme which neutralizes bradykinin, the natural substance that is formed by injured tissues and that is responsible for swelling and pain. This can account for the soothing effect of aloe juice upon superficial burns.

Magnesium lactate, another ingredient, blocks the formation of histamine, the natural substance formed by the body in response to allergic insults. That would explain why aloe can help to soothe poison ivy rashes and insect bites.

The plant also contains another anti-inflammatory compound that rather closely mimics the effects of aspirin and its newer variants (such as Motrin and Nuprin). This probably accounts for aloe juice's usefulness in certain types of long-standing dermatitis and as a healing promoter for certain ulcers (e.g: those due to varicose veins).

Last but not least, aloe contains anthroquinone, an irritant that accounts for its usefulness as a laxative and that, when applied to skin, is sometimes beneficial in psoriasis.

Depending upon where an aloe plant is grown, the amounts and proportions of these ingredients vary and, thus, it is likely that some plants will be better than others for specific purposes. Aloe on the skin, unfortunately, sometimes triggers a contact rash or an allergy. Such reactions are rare, however, and this is fortunate since aloe vera has become one of the most popular ingredients in cosmetics.

Baking Soda Baths for Itching

To relieve severe itching due to eczema, try soaking yourself for 10-15 minutes in a tub of warm water to which half a cupful of baking soda has been added, a letter to the editor of *Lancet* (2:977) suggests.

While this has not been mentioned in any of the medical textbooks, earlier correspondence in *Lancet* (2:464) reported that it is helpful for itching due to other causes. Baking soda is a lot less messy than some of the remedies traditionally recommended, such as oil, oatmeal, and coal tar. Other measures that can be helpful for itching include the avoidance of harsh soaps and detergents, and the maintenance of adequate humidity in the house during cold weather.

Since severe generalized itching is sometimes the symptom of thyroid disease, kidney trouble, liver disorders, and certain types of cancer, do not attempt to treat it yourself without first consulting your doctor.

Body Odor

Body odor is a common, distressing, and embarrassing problem that is not always easy to prevent, correspondence in the *Western Journal of Medicine* (146:367) reports.

In one case, an extremely foul body odor had suddenly developed and had persisted in spite of all attempts to control it with special soaps, extra bathing, and frequent changes of antiperspirant and deodorant.

On carefully reviewing this man's routine, his doctor discovered that he had recently started using Fresh Start laundry detergent, and suggested that he try another one. The man did so and was pleased to find that his odor problem immediately went away. Furthermore, now that he understood the problem, he was able to explain why his body odor returned not long after he had put on clothing which had been laundered with Fresh Start.

Obviously, the odor was produced by some kind of reaction occurring between his skin chemistry and the detergent residue in his clothes. Others with stubborn cases of B.O. might also wish to try using another detergent brand.

Bar Soap and Liquid Soap

Because soap bars become contaminated by the hands of the people who use them, they become reservoirs of bacteria, such as staphylococci, capable of causing boils and acne skin lesions, a letter to the editor of the *Journal of the American Medical Association* (253:1560) points out. Even when only one person uses the bar, bacteria can multiply upon it and cause no less trouble than if many people washed with it.

The gooey gel that forms under a wet bar of soap is usually the most contaminated part. This problem can be virtually eliminated if one uses a liquid or lotion soap instead of the bars. Kept in plastic dispensers, these soaps do not come in contact with the outside world.

STOMACH PROBLEMS

A Stomach Ulcer? Or is it Cancer?

One must be alert to the earliest symptoms of stomach cancer that distinguish it from peptic ulcer. These include weight loss with nausea, indigestion, and upper abdominal discomfort or pain right after meals. This timing is important, since simple peptic ulcer pain is usually relieved by food, while cancer pain tends to be brought on by meals, or is suddenly made worse by them.

Early stomach cancer produces pain similar to that of ordinary peptic ulcer, and we must be careful not to delay surgery (which can cure about one case in three) while we continue trying medications. The trap, according to the *British Medical Journal* (286:149) is that cancer pain may be largely relieved (at least temporarily) by antacids or the drug Cimetidine (Tagamet). Also, because so many gastric cancer patients have previously had a peptic ulcer, they may assume that a new bout of pain is merely a recurrence.

Quite apart from the danger that Cimetidine is masking stomach cancer symptons, there is also the possibility that Cimetidine may actually induce stomach cancer by reducing acidity and thereby permitting growth in the stomach of bacteria that form carcinogenic nitrosamines. People who are taking this drug should be aware of these dangers and consult their physicians at once if they have a question about symptoms.

Pain Drugs and the Stomach

Nowadays, most of the drugs used for arthritis and other types of moderate pain are non-steroidal anti-inflammatory drugs (NSAIDs), a group of agents that includes aspirin as well. While effective in relieving pain, NSAIDs are "two-edged swords" that cause a lot of side effects including even gastric ulcers in possibly up to 20 percent of patients who take them regularly for a long time.

Fortunately, the *American Family Physician* (32#4:275) reports, there is a new NSAID that is much less likely than all the others to injure the stomach. Named Salsalate, it is chemically very similar to aspirin, but lacks that acetic acid part of the molecule which makes aspirin so irritating to the stomach. Nonetheless, Salsalate is probably just as effective.

People who fail to respond to it will have to use one of the other NSAIDs. If in doing so they are likely to have a gastric problem, the stomach can be protected with an additional drug, such as Ranitidine, taken simultaneously to prevent acid secretion.

Coca-Cola and Stomach Acid

By drinking Coca-Cola, we significantly increase the amount of acid in the stomach and duodenum, the parts of the gastrointestinal tract that are most prone to ulceration, the journal *Gut* (25:386) reports. This could seriously interfere with the healing of peptic ulcers, could be responsible for their relapses and, the report suggests, may even predispose us to the development of ulcers.

In view of these findings, ulcer patients should avoid Coca-Cola. It may also be wise for people who have a peptic ulcer to avoid the many similar soft drinks, which could possibly have the same effect.

STROKES

Warning of Stroke

Transient ischemic attacks (TIA) are disturbances of brain function, usually lasting from two minutes to two hours, but sometimes for as long as 24 hours, which leave no trace. During a TIA, the victim may be paralyzed, unable to talk, or experience tingling or other unusual feelings on one side of the face or in one side of the body. There may also be dizziness, or partial loss of vision and hearing. One or more of these phenomena can occur repeatedly, or they may appear in different combinations from time-to-time, ranging from momentary dimming of vision to severe but temporary stroke-like attacks.

Caused by temporary blockage of arteries supplying the brain, TIAs often result from blood clots carried there from elsewhere in the body. A failing heart or a damaged heart valve is the usual site of the clot formation, but other conditions (including atherosclerosis, diabetes, or early tumors) may provide the stimulus for clotting. For this reason, anyone who begins having TIAs needs to be examined by a physician to determine whether medical or surgical treatment is required for an underlying disease.

Even when no underlying cause is found, TIA victims can benefit from continuous anticoagulant drug treatment to slow the clotting process. This treatment should be carefully monitored and changed at intervals to match the patient's varying needs. Regular follow-up visits to the doctor are therefore essential, even though one may feel perfectly well.

Aspirin for Stroke Prevention

It has been known for some time that a small daily dose of aspirin reduces the incidence of stroke. It does this by affecting certain types of our blood cells.

Blood cells are of three types: red cells (which carry oxygen), white cells (which defend us against infection), and platelets (plate-shaped cells that seal holes in blood vessels). Whenever there is bleeding, thousands of platelets settle at the site of the broken vessel to plug the hole. They also release a chemical that starts blood clotting at the site of injury. Drugs like aspirin, that "stabilize" platelets by slowing up their sealing and clotting activities, therefore cause increased bruising and more prolonged bleeding than would be expected after minor trauma.

On the good side, daily doses of aspirin can help to prevent clots from forming spontaneously inside blood vessels, thereby also helping to prevent stroke (due to clotting in an artery of the brain) and myocardial infarction (heart attack due to blocking of a coronary artery).

During a recent study in France, *Internal Medicine Alert* (5#3:11) reports, either a daily aspirin or placebo (the patients did not know which) was taken by patients who had experienced transient ischemic attacks (warning symptoms of stroke, such as episodes of slurred speech, weakness on one side, loss of vision, etc). Results were clear cut, with only 10 percent of the aspirin group developing stroke, as compared to 18 percent in the placebo group.

This French study confirmed earlier studies in the United States and Canada but differed from them in showing that aspirin can prevent strokes not only in men but also in women. This was an important contribution. Women are more likely to benefit equally with men when their aspirin dosage is reduced in proportion to their lower weight. One baby aspirin (about 100 mg) daily is probably enough.

Aspirin as a preventive treatment may be much more powerful than has so far been suspected. A Georgetown University neurologist who is an expert on this subject believes that, until now, researchers have focused too much upon the number of strokes that occur on various preventive regimens. More meaningful information can be obtained, he believes, when one studies the severity of strokes as well as their numbers.

Thus, *Modern Medicine* (26#12:8) reports, a daily aspirin reduces the severity of strokes even more than it reduces their number. Preliminary clinical studies even suggest that daily aspirin cuts the number of strokes that are severe (fatal ones or those that leave the victim paralyzed) by 80 percent. The strokes that occur on this regimen have usually been mild ones from which most of the victims have recovered fully. Additional studies are now is progress to determine if this exciting preliminary work can be confirmed.

TEETH

Mouthwash and the Teeth

Periodontal disease, manifested by gum shrinkage, is the main cause of tooth loss after the age of 40 and is principally due to accumulation of plaque on the roots of the teeth, the *U.S. Pharmacist* (10#9:23) reports. Plaque is a sticky, soft material composed of bacteria trapped within a gel-like mixture of mucus, broken-down cells, and debris from food. Left undisturbed, it gradually builds up and hardens, irritating and displacing the gums so that they shrink back from the teeth. Ultimately, this results in cavities, loosening and loss of teeth.

Apart from brushing after meals and using dental floss, procedures that cannot reach all of the bacteria that form plaque, most of us do nothing more to prevent plaque build-up than visiting our dentists for a tooth cleaning session about once a year.

Plaque formation can be much more effectively prevented if, in addition to doing all of the above, one uses a mouthwash containing chemicals such as cetylpyridinium and alcohol that inhibit growth of plaque-producing bacteria. One should rinse the mouth with about two tablespoonfuls of the liquid twice a day for about 30 seconds, swishing it around between the teeth before spitting it out. After rinsing, do not eat or drink for 30 minutes. Mouthwash is most effective when used immediately after brushing and, if used regularly, reduces plaque formation by about 70 percent.

Gums, Teeth and Vitamin C

Dietary experiments with monkeys have now clearly established that vitamin C helps to prevent inflammation and recession of the gums. Even when the vitamin C shortage is not severe enough to cause any other signs, normally harmless trauma leads to redness, swelling, bleeding and "pocket" formation of the gums around the roots of the teeth.

Of course, the *Journal of the American Medical Association* (246:730) points out, it has been known for hundreds of years that swollen, bleeding gums are major features of scurvy, the disease caused by a severe shortage of vitamin C. The importance of these new findings, however, is that unhealthy receding gums can result from such a minor shortage of vitamin C that it is hardly severe enough to be called a deficiency. The trouble is that once your gums have shrunk down to expose the roots of your teeth, no amount of supplementary vitamin or anything else can make them grow back again. Here is another good reason for taking extra vitamin C.

One must remember, however, that vitamin C is an acid (ascorbic acid) and is therefore capable of injuring the teeth, decalcifying, and eroding them when it stays in contact with them for any great length of time.

The *Journal of the American Dental Association* (107:253) reports the case of a 30-year-old woman that illustrates this danger very well. Several back teeth on one side of her mouth (the side on which she chewed) had become severely eroded and broken down, a condition that was readily understandable in view of her history of chewing three vitamin C tablets every day.

Chewable vitamin C, therefore, is best avoided by everyone except those who have a complete set of dentures, both lower and upper.

Denture Discomfort

Dentures cause pain not only when a rough spot rubs the gums but also when the tissues become irritated by or are allergic to one of the chemicals from which dentures are made, *Cutis* (36:384). Reactions of this kind are most likely when dentures are new or have just been repaired by addition of new material.

The best way of determining if allergy to a denture chemical is irritating the gum is for the dentist to make a button-sized disk of exactly the same acrylic material and tape it to the skin. The diagnosis is confirmed if the skin reacts as well.

Treatment of such reactions is very simple. All that the dentist need do, according to *Cutis*, is to put the dentures back in the hardening oven for another four hours to "double cure" them and then boil them gently for one hour. This heating drives off volatile chemicals that trigger reactions.

Bacteria in Toothbrushes

Lingering throat and mouth infections may be due to bacteria living in our toothbrushes, *Medical World News* (27#5:68) reports. This discovery was made by a professor of oral pathology after he compared bacteria on the brushes of 10 healthy people and 10 people with mouth and throat infections. The latter's infections quickly cleared up after he suggested that they start using new brushes every few weeks. It takes only 17-35 days, he discovered, for a new toothbrush to become heavily infected.

This is not surprising when one considers that tooth-brushes' provide a moist environment, are kept in warm bathrooms, and are regularly enriched with food from the mouth. Mouth infections may be easier to overcome, there-fore, if you change toothbrushes every few weeks.

TUMORS

A Cluster of Tumors in Texas

During a recent five-month period, the *Journal of the American Medical Association* (253:2843) reports, six children in a Texas rural community were affected by a rather rare lymph node cancer, known as Burkitt's tumor. Usually fatal, this tumor first appears in the neck, jaws or throat of its victims, but later spreads throughout the body.

Similar clustering of Burkitt's tumor cases, but on a larger scale, has been occurring for many years in Africa, where the Epstein-Barr virus (EBV), conveyed by mosquito bites, was discovered to be the cause. In Europe and in the U.S.A., EBV causes the common infectious disease, mononucleosis, and a long-lasting flu-like illness.

Why EBV only sometimes causes a cluster of cases of Burkitt's tumor (which does not appear to spread from person to person) remains unknown.

There is a plausible theory, however, that Burkitt's tumor results from the exceptionally heavy infection with EBV that occurs only when someone who is not yet immune to the virus, usually a child, gets bitten by a very large number of carrier mosquitoes at the same time. Several conditions must be met for this to occur including the climate, mosquitoes of the right species to carry EBV, and susceptible children who spend enough time outdoors to be heavily bitten.

One can only speculate that an African type of mosquito is now in Texas. If so, let us hope it does not spread. The moral of this story, therefore, is to use a good repellent and to keep the children indoors when mosquitoes are abundant.

One-Sided Breast Tumors

The Chinese "boat people" of Hong Kong, according to *Lancet*, traditionally feed their babies only from the right breast and, among their menopausal women who develop breast cancer, tumors are several times more common on the left side than the right. Other populations sometimes show a slight difference in breast tumor sidedness but never a great preponderance like this. Chinese boat people are unique.

The bad outcome of only using one breast is not surprising. A constantly engorged breast never empties and its secretions (including ingested and inhaled pollutants) remain forever trapped in the ducts of that breast, irritating them and in some cases, ultimately transforming them into tumor tissue. Bottle feeding does not carry the same risk as using only one breast because both breasts dry up quickly when neither one is used.

Fluorescent Light

In mice, at least, there seems to be a strong case against cool white fluorescent lighting. Investigators of the National Institute of Environmental Health Sciences have shown that mice of a certain cancer-prone strain develop tumors earlier in life if raised under fluorescent lighting. Reduced fertility was another effect encountered in these mice.

According to *Science 81* (2#6:7), this research confirms the suspicions of other scientists that fluorescent lighting may be harmful. For us humans, the big unanswered question is whether fluorescent lighting harms us too.

URINARY PROBLEMS

Urinary Incontinence in the Elderly

When elderly people become incontinent of urine, this is usually assumed to be permanent. Such pessimism, however, is unjustified since about 80-90 percent of these cases can be cured, the *Annals of Internal Medicine* (104:429) points out. Even the incontinence that follows a stroke can, in many instances, be overcome.

Before anything can be done, though, the patient must be seen by a physician who has special training (usually a geriatrician or urologist) to have the cause of the incontinence correctly determined. Some cases, of course, are "surgical" and can be cured with an operation for such things as prostate enlargement or a uterus that has slipped down out of place. For patients not needing surgery, treatment with an appropriate medicine, biofeedback, or habit training cures over 70 percent.

Older people whose incontinence is caused by muscular weakness can do a lot to help themselves with exercises that tone up the muscles of the pelvic floor. The exercises involved tightening and relaxing the muscles repeatedly for 15 minutes three times every day, the *U S Pharmacist* (12#8:92) reports. By stopping and starting the flow of urine, victims of incontinence can learn to identify those muscles that need to be strengthened. The same muscles control the passage of stools. Identical exercises, incidentally, are employed by women after childbirth to tone up muscles that support the uterus. To do any good, these exercises need to be performed three times every day for at least three months.

Victims of incontinence should be aware of the fact that both constipation and alcohol can interfere with the function of the pelvic floor muscles. They should also avoid drinking coffee, tea and grapefruit juice, all of which can suddenly increase the need to pass more urine. Cranberry juice is a useful substitute.

In addition, they should routinely empty the bladder before and after every meal and at bedtime, even if they feel no need to do so. They should always respond promptly to the urge to urinate, and must never ignore it. In a few cases, surgical repair may be required, especially if the bladder has become displaced by repeated childbirth or by removal of the prostate

VITAMIN, MINERAL DOSAGES

What is "Vitamin B15"?

In the United States, it is illegal to sell "vitamin B15"

(pangamic acid, calcium pangamate), and according to the *Journal of the American Medical Association* (243:2473), the FDA is prosecuting distributors who handle it and are seizing it from health food stores. Furthermore, the courts are backing up FDA's right to destroy the materials they have seized.

Not just playing cops and robbers, the FDA is truly worried by the fact that two of the most widely available brands of this "vitamin" were found to contain substances which, after being swallowed, turn into some of the most potent cancer-producing chemicals known.

Even worse, different brands have been found to have completely different compositions so that the terms vitamin B15 and pangamate are meaningless. Pangamate, incidentally, is derived from the Greek words pan, meaning all, and gamete, meaning seed, and has been applied to mixtures of substances extracted from all kinds of seeds.

Furthermore, it is not a "vitamin" in the usual sense of the word since it has never been shown to be an essential dietary ingredient and there has been no definition of its chemical nature.

"Producers can throw anything they want into a bottle and label it vitamin B15 or pangamic acid," reports the *Journal,* and producers have alleged that it helps heart disease, aging, diabetes, hypertension, glaucoma, alcoholism, hepatitis, jaundice, allergies, neuralgia, and neuritis.

Vitamin A Overdose

Of late, vitamin A has been much in the news as a drug that reduces the incidence of certain cancers. Accordingly, for the sake of fair balance, we felt that our readers should be told about a recent report in the *Western Journal of Medicine*

(137:429).

A young woman visited her doctor because dryness of the eyes made it uncomfortable for her to wear her contacts. She also complained of a sore tongue and gums, cracking of the skin at the corners of the mouth, and generalized itching and dryness of the skin. She also had a continuous headache, felt nauseated, and had frequently vomited during the previous seven days. Devoted to jogging, she nevertheless had had to give it up because of severe pains in her bones.

On being questioned in the hospital, this lady (a health food store employee) admitted taking 25,000 units of vitamin A daily (five times the "recommended daily allowance") for several months. Tests showed abnormally high vitamin A blood levels that, among other things, had disturbed her liver. All of these signs and symptoms were typical of toxicity due to excess of vitamin A.

Treatment with intravenous fluids normalized this woman's blood levels of vitamin A in about a week. Had she taken vitamin A in excess for much longer, however, early death from liver failure would have become inevitable. The lesson, then, is to take only enough vitamin A to avoid deficiency and bolster resistance against cancer, the recommended daily allowance (RDA), but do not take it in excess.

Excess Vitamin A in Liver Dishes

Since liver has the reputation of being an inexpensive but "complete" food, dishes employing it are often recommended for dieters who wish to eat sparingly but well.

Regardless of one's reason for eating a lot of liver, the danger is the same — it can provide too much vitamin A. Because liver is an animal's storehouse for vitamin A, we can acquire much more of it than we can handle if we eat a lot of liver nearly every day.

In extreme cases, when hungry explorers have eaten nearly all of the liver of a shark or of a polar bear, both of which contain exceptional amounts of vitamin A (many thousands of times the recommended daily allowance for humans), sudden death from brain swelling has occurred. In the more usual cases, when people have eaten beef or chicken liver several times a week, the illness is much less dramatic.

Typically, *Emergency Medicine* (17#8:105) reports, the symptoms of milder and more usual cases of vitamin A intoxication include long-lasting headaches and blurring of vision. Victims also sometimes complain of a momentary loss or sudden dimming of vision lasting but a second or two.

Another fairly common symptom is a pulsating swishing or ringing noise in the ears. There may also be nausea and vomiting in some cases, but these symptoms are less common and occur, in addition to the other symptoms mentioned above, only when the blood vitamin A level suddenly rises even further above normal following ingestion of a vitamin tablet.

Proof of this diagnosis is simple and involves simply taking a blood sample and sending it to the laboratory for measurement of the vitamin A level. Since prevention is better than cure, avoid this problem by eating liver only in modera-tion. For instance, giving a baby a can of ground chicken liver every day might well provide him with too much

Vitamin B6 Toxicity

Vitamin B6 (also known as pyridoxine) became "front page news" when it was discovered that, in megadoses, it causes such serious nerve damage and difficulty in walking that people have had to give up their jobs.

It has been thought that pyridoxine nerve damage would occur only with daily doses in the range of 2000-6000 mg (two to six grams), or 1000 times the recommended daily allowance (RDA) of two to four mg. Now, however, according to correspondence in the *New England Journal of Medicine* (311:986), it has even taken place in an otherwise healthy young woman who took only 500 mg every day. After 12 months on this dosage, she experienced shooting pa ns and increasing numbness in her limbs, and such difficulty in balancing on her feet that it became impossible to walk unaided in the dark or with her eyes closed. These are typical of the symptoms experienced by people who have been taking megadoses of vitamin B6. Brief exposure to very high dosage therefore appears to have the same toxic effect as longer exposure to doses of a more moderate size. Either way, the dosage involved have always been a few hundred times larger than the RDA. Consumers need to be alert to this danger since 500 mg tablets of vitamin B6 can still be purchased without a doctor's prescription.

Like all other "water-soluble" vitamins, vitamin B6 has traditionally been considered harmless, regardless of the dosage. This experience, however, shows that in megadoses it is definitely unsafe.

After normal doses of pyridoxine (two to four milligrams daily), the body converts it into pyridoxal phosphate, the "active" form of vitamin B6. Pyridoxal phosphate is then taken up by the tissues and becomes a part of many enzymes (the cnemical "machinery" of cells).

The *Journal* speculates that the body is chemically so overwhelmed by megadoses of pyridoxine that it cannot convert more than a small fraction of it into the active phosphate form. Unaltered pyridoxine, it goes on to suggest, then floods the tissues in such abundance that the cells take it up instead of the phosphate. In this way, the excess of plain pyridoxine could block the cells' enzymes and prevent them from taking up the small normal amounts of pyridoxal phosphate still available.

Alternatively, the *Journal* suggests, manufactured pyridoxine may contain small amounts of a poisonous impurity. Normal doses of pyridoxine would not provide sufficient impurity to do harm, but in megadoses, the amount of impurity could be dangerous. Either way, pyridoxine in daily doses 100-1000 greater than the RDA of two to four mg has proved to be very toxic. Taking 100-1000 times the usual dose of almost anything might be expected to cause trouble, and megadosing, in general, seems to be a rather risky fad.

Vitamin B6 and Birth Defects

Pyridoxine (vitamin B6), a letter in the *Lancet* (1:636) suggests, may be like Thalidomide in its ability to cause human birth defects. The letter reports the birth of a child with nearly total absence of the right lower leg, the type of defect seen so often in babies whose mothers, during pregnancy, had taken Thalidomide.

By itself, this report would not be sufficient to incriminate pyridoxine as the cause of birth defects (it could have been a coincidence), but viewed in the context of pyridoxine's other known side effects, it looks highly suspicious. Given repeatedly in large enough doses, both Thalidomide and pyridoxine, it has been found, cause almost the same type of nerve damage in the limbs, with numbness and tingling in the "stocking and glove" areas, progressing to weakness and instability in walking.

This suggests that pyridoxine and Thalidomide share a common toxic effect on human tissue, and that this is also capable of producing birth defects. Although there is no proof of this, it would be prudent to avoid the current fad of taking supplemental pyridoxine.

The woman whose baby was deformed, incidentally, had been taking one 50 mg tablet of pyridoxine every day.

Vitamin E Overdosage

Claimed by enthusiasts as an anti-aging vitamin and as a remedy for most skin disorders, vitamin E is not considered effective for these purposes by most doctors and dietitians. They agree, however, that it helps tissues defend themselves against harmful oxidant "free radicals" that may be one cause of cancer.

However, for that, one needs no more vitamin E than the Recommended Daily Allowance (RDA), which is 10 mg daily for a large man. More than this does harm, and *Geriatrics* (39#2:69) lists the signs and symptoms that usually result from excessive dosage.

The most serious side effects include: thrombophlebitis (inflammation and tenderness under the skin, with bumps and bruises over the veins), pulmonary embolism (blood clots lodging in the circulation of the lung, causing a dangerous illness, with pain in the chest, shortness of breath and blood spitting), high blood pressure, severe fatigue, and tender enlargement of the breasts. Some more easily seen effects include: chapped lips, sore mouth, blister-like rashes, and very slow healing of wounds. Others are: nausea, diarrhea, intestinal cramps, and night blindness (due to vitamin A deficiency since very large doses of vitamin E antagonize vitamin A).

Since vitamin E capsules containing several times the RDA are on sale, many people must be taking it in dangerously large amounts. The *Journal of the American Medical Association* (246:129) recently published an article deploring the fashionable habit of taking vitamin E in "megadoses" every day and reported that the author sees many patients with the side effects of overdosage with vitamin E.

Unfortunately, the cause of its bad effects can easily be overlooked since they rarely all appear together or begin until large doses have been taken for many months.

Vitamin D Excess

Softening of children's bones with permanent bowing of the legs, ("bandy legs"), medically known as rickets, was fairly common before World War II. With the discovery that rickets is caused by vitamin D deficiency, bandy legs have become rare.

Now, with rickets a thing of the past, physicians are beginning to see an illness due to vitamin D excess called hypercalcemia, a high concentration of calcium in the blood. Symptoms of hypercalcemia include weakness, nausea, vomiting, thirst, frequent urination, and distaste for food. Left untreated, hypercalcemia can produce kidney stones and kidney damage with high blood pressure.

According to the *Lancet* (1: 229), people vary in the amount of vitamin D excess they can tolerate without getting hypercalcemia, and it may not be safe for everyone to take a tablet containing vitamin D every day. The elderly who are not eating well and all growing children probably can benefit from taking a multi-vitamin tablet (containing vitamin D) every day, but well-nourished adults usually get enough vitamin D from their food, unless they are on a diet.

Zinc Deficiency

Zinc, it is now well understood, is no less essential for good nutrition than other minerals, such as calcium and iron. Signs of zinc deficiency include an impaired sense of taste, dry skin, falling hair, and wounds that are slow to heal. In children, zinc deficiency can stunt growth and interfere with sexual maturation.

Zinc deficiency occurs most commonly in children (who may not get enough dietary zinc to allow for growth) and in the very old (who may not eat enough animal protein, the richest source of zinc). Furthermore, *Medical World News* (24#3:41) reports, since zinc deficiency dulls the appetite by reducing the sense of taste, zinc deficient persons eat less and become even more short of zinc. The extreme of this condition is the anorexia nervosa patient, and we discuss the important role of zinc for this disorder in the article, "Zinc and Anorexia Nervosa," in the section *Anorexia Nervosa*.

Zinc deficiency is also very likely to be found in pregnant women, even among those who are eating well. The reason for this paradox, it seems, is twofold. First, the demands of growth require the pregnant woman to provide the fetus with extra zinc, and secondly, this may be occurring at a time when the mother's ability to absorb zinc is reduced.

Zinc deficiency is understandably a concern for vegetarians since vegetables contain very little zinc and meat is very rich in it. In addition, soy protein and vegetable fiber tightly bind with zinc, holding it in the intestines and stopping it from being absorbed.

A surgical operation or an acute infection (i.e., a cold or the flu), can suddenly bring on signs of zinc deficiency in persons whose status is already borderline. Chronic diarrhea, chronic infection (i.e., tuberculosis), and sickle cell deficiency also increase our need for zinc.

Iron, according to the *British Medical Journal* (287:1013), when taken together with zinc, competes with zinc for absorption and significantly reduces the amount of zinc that the body is able to retain. Therefore, it seems, it is not efficient to take iron and zinc together, and it is probably better to take them at different times of day, spaced as far as possible apart. What the optimal spacing of these doses might be yet remains to be worked out. It has also been pointed out that, for similar reasons, iron and calcium also should be taken at different times of day.

Dietary zinc is naturally obtained from meat and other high cost protein foods, and for this reason, zinc deficiency is seen more commonly in times of economic stress.

For any of the above reasons, you may be considering taking a zinc supplement. Before you do, read the next article on zinc overdosage, since that can cause problems too.

Zinc Overdosage

As noted in the previous article, there are many factors which could contribute to a zinc deficiency, and concerned people will want to make sure they take enough of this important mineral. However, zinc taken regularly in doses greater than three times the minimum daily requirement, according to the *American Family Physician* (26#2:167), can easily do more harm than good. Thus, for the average person, one capsule daily of 220 mg of zinc sulfate is more than enough and should not be continued for very long.

Too much zinc produces liver disease, with lethargy, upper abdominal pain and fever, and displaces other metals from the body (producing anemia, etc.). It is important, therefore, to avoid taking extra zinc as a supplement unless one really needs it.

Contents of Zinc Tablets

Though zinc currently has great popularity as a dietary supplement, there is surprising confusion about the strengths of the various types of zinc tablets now being sold. In an attempt to learn exactly how much zinc (as the element) there is in each type of tablet and capsule being marketed in health food stores and drug stores (where they can only repeat what is on the labels), the author called several manufacturers. Confusion was the only consistent finding. Most of them, who are merely repackagers, stated that they had no exact knowledge of the nature of their zinc products since they buy the crystalline powder from a chemical manufacturer.

Perhaps the biggest obstacle to a proper understanding of the problem was their lack of knowledge as to how much water is included, along with the zinc salts (sulfate or gluconate) in the crystalline powders from which the tablets and capsules are made. Eventually, one of the largest manufacturers put some of its research staff to work on the problem and, after about 10 days, came up with a definite answer. They told us that one 220 mg tablet or capsule of zinc gluconate contains 28 mg of zinc and that one 100 mg tablet or capsule of zinc sulfate contains 22.5 mg of zinc.

The Recommended Daily Allowance (RDA) of zinc, according to Goodman and Gilmann's *The Pharmacological Basis of Therapeutics* (6th ed., p. 1553), is 15 mg. This amount, approximately, would be provided by one 110 mg tablet of zinc gluconate or by one 50 mg tablet of zinc sulfate. This much, it is believed, should be sufficient to maintain normal persons in a positive balance of zinc. Greater amounts than this, obviously, would be required to repair a deficiency state.

Calcium Supplements

Although bone meal (ground animal bones) would seem to be the most logical source of calcium for keeping our bones healthy and strong, it contains significant quantities of lead. This is understandable, the *U.S. Pharmacist* (8#3:27) comments, since lead in the soft tissues is poisonous and the body combats this danger by storing it away in the bones where it becomes biologically inert. Because there is always some lead in the environment, the older animals become, the more lead there is to be found in their bones. For this reason, the FDA advises, bone meal should be used sparingly if at all.

Dolomite is a calcium-bearing ground-up rock that also contains lead, but much less than there is to be found in bone meal. Even so, it can be toxic, especially for children, who are much more susceptible than are adults to poisoning by lead.

To be safe, it is therefore advisable to use pure salts of calcium (such as calcium carbonate, calcium lactate or calcium gluconate) that we can depend upon to be lead-free. Used as a supplement to maintain the integrity of the bones, calcium carbonate needs to be taken in doses of two to three tablets (each of 650 mg) daily. Only about 30 percent of the weight of each tablet is calcium: the rest is carbonate. In calcium lactate and gluconate tablets, the proportion of calcium is even less and, to get enough calcium, one must take several of them every day. Nevertheless, many people prefer them.

Used as antacids, calcium carbonate products are safer, no less effective, and considerably cheaper than aluminum-containing medications.

Sudden Folic Acid Deficiency in the Critically Ill

Although people in good health need only about 50 micrograms of folic acid every day, the need for this important member of the vitamin B complex increases dramatically (seven to 20-fold) during bacterial infections and after loss of blood. Extra folic acid is used whenever new cells are formed in large numbers anywhere in the body.

Thus, when the bone marrow produces many extra white blood cells to fight an infection or forms many new red blood cells to make up for blood lost during surgery or hemorrhage, it suddenly uses much more folic acid than usual. If this increased need is not recognized and met, the patient will be unable to produce all the necessary white cells, red cells, and platelets, or to recover completely from a serious infection, even though transfusions and antibiotics are employed.

A report in *Critical Care Medicine* (8:500) points out that during a serious illness, the bone marrow uses up its folic acid stores so fast that it becomes deficient in this essential vitamin even though folic acid levels in the blood and other tissues remain normal.

It may not be possible for patients to obtain all the vitamins they need by mouth when they are seriously ill, and to facilitate recovery, daily injections of folic acid (10 milligrams) may be required. Another reason that folic acid in tablet form may not be recommended, the *American Family Physician* (32#4:290) reports, is that it may cause a deficiency of zinc. If present in the stomach to excess, it is thought, folic acid combines with all of the zinc contained in our food, thus rendering it insoluble and less easily absorbed.

Foods such as peanut butter, beans, nuts, liver, and green leafy vegetables are natural sources of folic acid.

Selenium Toxicity

Since there is now good evidence that deficiency of selenium in our diet encourages the development of cancer, many people are taking supplementary selenium in the form of a tablet every day. One must be careful not to take too much selenium, however, since it can be very toxic if taken in excess.

Morbidity and Mortality Weekly Report (33:157) contains the story of a 57-year-old woman who took one selenium tablet daily and, after 11 days of this dosage, began losing her hair and developed sore fingertips. Continuing with the selenium because, at the time, she did not know that is was causing her problems, she slowly lost all of her hair during the next two months and developed a discharge around her nails, all of which she later lost as well. In addition, she suffered with episodes of nausea and vomiting, a sour-milk breath odor, and increasingly severe fatigue.

Eventually, her doctor found that her selenium blood level was four times higher than normal, and that this, in turn, was due to the selenium tablets being more than 100 times stronger than advertised.

The tablets (now recalled from the market) had been distributed in 15 states coast to coast. Knowing what to look out for, we should be able to quickly recognize selenium overdosage and protect ourselves against this danger.

Salt Substitute Danger

Salt substitutes contain potassium chloride in place of sodium chloride (our common table salt). Although by no means a "poison," potassium chloride must be used sparingly, otherwise too much potassium will get into the blood and tissues.

If it accumulates in the body to excess, a letter to *Journal of the American Medical Association* (256:1726) points out, muscle weakness and heart beat disturbances with, eventually, complete stoppage of the heart, can occur. The chances of potassium toxicity developing increase when someone using a salt substitute is also taking medicine for arthritis, heart failure or high blood pressure.

The *Journal*, for example, tells of a lady who had been taking medicines for angina pectoris (chest pains due to narrowing of the heart's coronary blood vessels) and had been consuming large quantities of homemade soup seasoned with salt substitute in place of regular salt. She became weak, could not stand, and complained of breathlessness and strange sensations in her limbs. In the hospital, she was found to have potassium intoxication, from which she was rescued with difficulty.

Although the labeling of salt substitutes (Morton's Lite Salt, Morton's Salt Substitute, Adolf's Salt Substitute, No-Salt, Nu-Salt) warns the consumer that they should never be used without the advice of a physician, they can be purchased from supermarkets without a doctor's prescription. Few people, therefore, are likely to take the warning seriously.

Furthermore, since salt is known to be dangerous for those with high blood pressure or heart failure, salt substitute products are generally thought of positively rather than negatively so far as their effects on health are concerned. Obviously, the public must be made more aware of the potential harm that can be done by salt substitutes.

WEIGHT LOSS

Obesity and Survival

Until recently, most doctors agreed that thin people are more likely to live longer than those who are even slightly overweight.

In the past few years, however, many experts have suggested that it is actually healthier for middle-aged people to put on some weight and not to stay as slim as they were during their most active early adult years. It was even suggested that new "ideal weight" tables be developed allowing people to put on about 10 pounds in each decade because certain statistics show that thin people have a higher death rate than those of average or slightly heavier weight.

Because of these conflicting viewpoints, the *Journal of the American Medical Association* (267:353) reports, a group of researchers at Harvard University Medical School has carefully analyzed all studies of this topic.

Their conclusion is that the thinner you are (if you are not thin because of an illness or smoking), the longer you are likely to live. They discovered, furthermore, that the reason why some people had begun to believe otherwise was that many recent weight/survival studies were carelessly conducted and statistically flawed.

It was found, for instance, that no attempt had been made to eliminate smokers and sick people from those studies, and that these were the people who tended to weigh less and to die earlier than the others. When these people's data were removed from the statistics, it became obvious that the lowest death rates occur in people who keep their weight to at least 10 pounds under the average for their age and height. The idea that it is beneficial to increase one's weight in middle age cannot be supported.

A significant increase in the coronary heart disease death rate is seen when people are 30 percent over their ideal weight, *Modern Medicine* (53#6:49) reports. Such "morbid obesity" increases the mortality from heart disease by 12 times in people aged 25-35, six times in those aged 35-45, and three times in those who are over 45.

Two Types of Obesity

Overweight people with big abdomens are in much worse health than are equally obese people whose fat is distributed around the hips and limbs, *Medical World News* (26#3:74) reports.

In people who are equally overweight, abdominal obesity carries about five times as much risk of heart attack and stroke as does fat deposited elsewhere. Fat in the abdomen, apparently, is much more "active", so far as the body's chemistry is concerned, than fat elsewhere. It is associated with elevation of the blood cholesterol levels, sluggishness of fat disposal by the liver, and impairment of insulin secretion in response to sugary meals.

The easiest way to determine a fat person's degree of risk from this type of obesity, according to the *News*, is to measure the circumferences both the waist and hips. When the waist-to-hips ratio is above 1.0 in men, or above 0.8 in women, the risk of heart attack and stroke is five to 10 times greater than normal.

Men, it has been found, are more prone than women to abdominal obesity, even though in general, they are less likely to be overweight. Beer drinkers had better beware.

Exercise and Weight Loss

A physically active lifestyle or hard exercise taken regularly every day make losing weight and staying slim very much easier. According to *Science Digest* (94#4:41), these beneficial effects are due to the fact that muscular activity burns up the body's fat stores while at the same time increasing the bulk of its muscles.

Muscle is a much more active tissue than fat and, pound for pound, has more cells and needs more calories just to maintain itself. Thus, people who have replaced fat with muscle develop a much more active metabolism that burns up more calories at rest and helps them to stay slim.

Dieting without exercise, on the other hand, results in loss of both fat and muscle tissue, and when the dieting is over, lost weight is quickly regained. Worse yet, weight regained under these circumstances is mostly due to fat. Cyclic loss and gain of weight due to dieting without exercise results in a new loss of muscle tissue that makes slimness even more difficult to attain in the future.

Dieting and Weight Loss

To be lastingly effective, weight-losing diets should be gradual and realistic and must never involve the omission of any meals. If one skips breakfast or any other meal, the body merely stores more of the calories from the next meals in the form of fat to make up for the period of fasting and, at the same time, decreases energy expenditure by one means or another (making one feel tired and sleep more).

Fasting is therefore not usually helpful for those who wish to lose weight. Rather, they should eat three meals a day at specified times, take predetermined amounts of food, eat slowly, and keep food out sight between meals.

One interesting study about dieting and weight loss did not emphasize quantity of food at all, but rather zeroed in on when the food was eaten. Even though the participants did not eat any less than usual, merely by doing most of their eating earlier in the day, these overweight people easily managed to lose five to 10 pounds every month, *Postgraduate Medicine* (79#4:352) reports.

The dietary research from which this finding emerged involved 595 overweight people treated in the Department of Nutrition at Tulane University's School of Public Health in New Orleans.

These people were instructed to change their eating patterns from heavy meals in the evening to a heavy morning meal, a modest lunch and a light afternoon snack, with no change in the daily total intake. They were also told not to go to sleep for at least eight and a half hours after the last meal of the day.

The report stressed that this was a "preliminary" finding that needs to be confirmed by studies involving a "control" comparison group treated some other way. Meanwhile, many who are feeling desperate about obesity will no doubt want to give this method a personal trial.

Drugs and Weight Loss

Drugs, such as thyroid, amphetamines, human chorionic gonadotropin, and phenylpropanolamine (an appetite suppressant), cautions *Postgraduate Medicine* (72#1:121), do not have any lasting effect and are therefore not useful in slimming and long-term weight control. Drugs expose one needlessly to the hazard of side effects and also involve considerable expense.

Four women, all of whom had been taking over-the-counter appetite suppressant pills containing the drug phenylpropanolamine (PPA) to lose weight, were recently admitted at various times to the same hospital with severe headache, clouding of consciousness, and inability to move parts of their bodies. A brain hemorrhage proved to be the diagnosis in every case, and the outcome was death for two of them.

PPA is similar to amphetamine and shares its ability to elevate the blood pressure (BP). In some people, PPA also injures the arteries, making them fragile and prone to leak, particularly if the BP rises above normal as well. When bleeding occurs inside the head, as it did in the four women reported by the *Western Journal of Medicine* (142:688), even neurosurgery may not help if many arteries are fragile and leaking.

Other brain side effects caused by PPA include anxiety,

psychosis and convulsions. Furthermore, when arteries in other parts of the body are affected, the organs supplied by them will also suffer. Thus, PPA usage has been associated with abnormal heart rhythms, heart attacks, kidney failure, and perforation of the intestines.

Perhaps the most disturbing aspect of so many PPA-associated adverse reactions is that they have occurred with dosages of the drug little if any above that normally recommended for curbing the appetite.

Surgery and Weight Loss

Because of the operative mortality (about 1 percent), surgical treatment for obesity should be undertaken only for emergency medical reasons (e.g., hypertension, uncontrolled diabetes, severe arthritis), and when the person is at least 100 pounds over ideal weight. Only under circumstances such as these can the risk of surgery be justified, since the risk of operating would then be less than that of not losing a lot of weight almost immediately.

Dramatic weight loss after an operation that reduces the size of the stomach sometimes also severely disturbs the emotions. This side effect of the surgery, the *American Journal of Gastroenterology* (78:321) reports, is sometimes caused by deficiency of vitamins of the B group which, like other foods, are no longer so well absorbed following the operation. Nervous system and brain functions depend upon absorption of normal amounts of the vitamin B complex.

With this in mind, the *Journal* suggests, anyone rapidly losing weight, whether because of dieting or surgery, must take a vitamin supplement that includes the B complex. No megadoses, please!

Salt and Obesity

Australian researchers at the University of Sydney have uncovered a most startling correlation between the amount of food we absorb after meals and their salt content, the *British Medical Journal* (292:1697) reports.

Until now, it was believed that the only way in which salt could increase our weight was by causing more water to be held in the tissues. The Australian discovery, however, suggests that salt's role in increasing body weight could be much more enduring.

After a starchy meal (i.e., lentils or bread), one can show that the blood sugar level rises to a certain height for a certain time, and that both of these things depend upon the size of the meal. Thus, the larger the meal, the higher the blood sugar level rises and the longer it takes for it to fall back down to normal again.

Such blood sugar "curves" following a standard-sized starchy meal are ordinarily very reproducible. The Australians, however, have shown that even without increasing the amount of starch in the meal, one can nevertheless increase both the height and duration of the blood sugar curve resulting from it, if one takes salt with the food.

Salt, therefore, either boosts digestion of food in the intestine so that more sugar is released from it, or it stimulates the intestine to absorb sugar more efficiently. Either way, salt makes more calories become available to the body from the same amount of food.

These findings strongly suggest that if we wish to be slim, we need to carefully limit the amount of salt that we take in our food. While this could be important for any of us, it is more so for diabetics, especially if they have been experiencing inexplicably high levels of blood sugar despite a carefully controlled diet. This research, of course, needs to be confirmed, but that should not be a difficult task.

Born to be Fat?

A clue to why some of us can stay trim on a diet that causes others to gain weight may be found in the way the body handles sodium and potassium.

According to a recent report in *Science News* (118:295), Harvard Medical researchers have found there is a direct relationship between body weight and the capacity to move sodium and potassium through body membranes. Since this transport process burns up a lot of energy, a relative lack of sodium and potassium transporters could understandably be associated with increased body weight.

"For the first time we have evidence that obese people have a primary biochemical defect not caused by overeating," reported one of the researchers. The question of whether the biochemical defect is hereditary remains to be fully answered. Meanwhile, let us not use this as an excuse. It may be harder for some of us to diet if we have fewer than normal sodium and potassium transporters, but it is not impossible.

Water-Induced Seizures

A weight loss organization with over 650 centers throughout the U.S.A., Canada, and Germany urges its patrons to drink at least eight to 12 glasses of water every day, and even possibly more, as part of its program, a letter to the editor of *New England Journal of Medicine* (312:246) reports.

The writer of the letter, a Stanford University Medical

School physician, had three patients with a recent recurrence of epileptic seizures. All three were epileptics but, with medication, had been seizure-free for many years.

They began to have seizures again after drinking more water, as recommended by the weight loss organization. Since excessive hydration is known to bring on seizures, especially in those who are already prone to them, drinking eight to 12 glasses of water a day cannot safely be recommended for everybody.

A good rule is to drink enough so that one produces about a quart of pale urine every day. If one does not drink enough, the urine becomes dark and too scanty. Of course, depending upon the climate, one's temperature, and how much one sweats, even more than 12 glasses of water a day might sometimes be needed.

Jogging and Overweight

Overweight people trying to shed pounds would be wiser not to do so by jogging. Bones and joints in the legs and feet can be severely stressed by this type of exercise when one is overweight. The combination of running and excess weight can even crack the bones of the pelvis in otherwise fit young people, according to *Medical World News* (23#25:57). The cracked bone causes aching in the buttock with hip movements, and requires that, for six weeks, all activities that produce the pain be stopped.

Exercise can certainly help dieters. However, it should be of a kind that does not overly stress weight-bearing structures in the lower limbs. Walking three or four miles a day or working up a sweat on an exercycle or rowing machine is helpful and safe. It is better to lose weight by other means first before taking up running or jogging.

WELLNESS, FITNESS

Fitness or Good Health?

By working out strenuously every day, one becomes fit but not necessarily healthy, the *Physician and Sportsmedicine* (11#6:156) points out.

Fitness is the ability to perform such feats as running a four-minute mile, while healthiness means being able to remain comfortably active well into old age.

To be healthy, one must engage in activity, such as walking the dog for a few miles, always using stairs rather than elevators, even just gardening, regularly every day. Health, of course, also involves such things as not smoking, having a sensibly balanced diet, and not letting one's waistline grow too large.

Remember, those who are fit are not necessarily healthy as well, and may bring on arthritis or develop heart attacks by running. Obviously, it is best to be both healthy and fit, which is possible if one starts working toward these goals early enough in life and does not overdo the strenuous exercise.

However, if one must choose between them, health is more desirable than fitness. Nowadays, as more and more people give up jogging, it is important for them to continue with regular health-promoting activities instead.

Is Jogging Safe?

Every year, just enough slim young people collapse and die while jogging that many physicians hesitate to recommend this form of exercise. At autopsy, the heart muscle in these cases usually looks as if it has not been getting enough blood supply. Until recently, however, the cause of this has been a mystery, since the young victims' coronary arteries are rarely found to be narrowed by fat and cholesterol deposits (atherosclerosis).

Now, it seems, the mystery has been solved by the discovery of "bridges" of heart muscle across the coronary arteries. When the muscle contracts, the bridges squeeze the coronary arteries and thus reduce the amount of blood they can deliver to the heart muscle. Since the bridges are part of the heart's muscular wall, coronary blood flow is reduced most severely during exercise when the heart is beating faster and more forcibly than usual. There could be no worse time for this to happen.

Since few of us know whether or not we have this abnormality (only 1 percent of us do), it is recommended that we avoid exercising our hearts past the point where bridges, if present, would tighten excessively around our vessels.

According to a report in *Medical World News,* this means not letting your pulse rate exceed 150 per minute. If your pulse beats faster than this during exercise, rest until it slows down and thereafter exercise more slowly. By training, you will more easily be able to keep your pulse below 150.

Leg and lower body exercise, as in jogging, has become a national compulsion which, as the body ages, may do more harm than good, the editorial writer in *Modern Medicine* suspects. The trauma of repeatedly pounding one's feet on pavement while jogging, he points out, damages the ankles, knees, hips, and spine because the human body (unlike the bodies of four-legged animals) is just not well designed for endurance running.

Should Children Run with Their Parents?

The answer, according to *Journal of the American Medical Association* (255:850), is definitely no. Preadolescents are less able than adults to lose excess heat from the body when they become overheated and, accordingly, can harm themselves in trying to keep up with their parents on long distance runs.

Heat stroke and heart damage, consequently, are more likely to occur. Also, there are "growth plates" at the end of children's bones that can be injured by the repetitive jarring that occurs during long runs, producing stress fractures that can be permanently disabling.

Do not invite your child to join you in long distance running, therefore, until he or she is past puberty.

Good News for Low-Mileage Joggers

Lack of exercise lets our muscles become flabby, permits the blood fats to rise, and thereby worsens atherosclerosis (hardening of the arteries). This, in turn, causes earlier deaths from high blood pressure, heart disease, and stroke.

Measurable improvement in the blood fats occurs when people exercise regularly. Surprisingly, people who run only about a mile a day (or two miles three times a week) show the same beneficial changes in their blood fats as those who run in marathons.

So, "Even moderate exercise is beneficial because ...it has a protective effect," writes a professor of physical medicine in *Physician and Sportsmedicine*. To be helpful, exercise should be taken at least three times a week. Exercising only once or twice weekly is not enough.

Runners' Iron Needs

Rather than improving their health by regular long-distance running, teenagers may eventually make themselves unwell, feeling constantly weak and tired and less able to do well in competitive sports, the *American Journal of Diseases of Children* (139:1115) reports.

These are the effects of iron deficiency. Iron is needed in our tissues (particularly by the muscles) and not merely in our red blood cells. However, when there is an iron shortage in the body, its level in the tissues falls first and before the blood is affected by anemia. Thus, despite feeling weak as the result of iron deficiency, a teen-age runner may not yet have become pale and anemic.

Special tests can demonstrate this shortage of iron in the tissues. Iron is lost from the body during long-distance running because a certain amount of blood (which contains a lot of iron) always leaks into the intestines while they are being repeatedly jarred by the excessive movement. Some iron also leaves the body through the skin during heavy sweating. Often, improper food that contains too much sugar and starch but not enough iron makes matters worse.

Correction of this type of deficiency is easily accomplished with iron tablets (525 mg of ferrous sulfate daily), taken with vitamin C to enhance its absorption. First, however, the runner should see a physician to rule out more serious causes of weakness. If iron deficiency is the cause, its correction quickly restores a runner's ability to compete. Otherwise, do not take any extra iron.

Longevity of Orchestra Conductors

Who lives longer, joggers or orchestra conductors? The answer, according to an editorial in *Modern Medicine* (53#2:21) is that, in this country at least, one hears of many more conductors, virtuoso violinists, and concert pianists than sportsmen not only living to a very ripe old age, but also remaining on the job right up to the end. Eubi Blake, 100; Karl Boehm, 86; Adrian Boult, 100; Arthur Fiedler, 86; Paul Paray, 93; Arthur Rubinstein, 94; Arturo Toscanini, 90; Walter Demrosch, 85; and Leopold Stokowski, 96, are a few examples.

How musicians manage to live such long and active lives is not understood, at least not from any scientifically-proven point of view.

Nevertheless, it is widely believed that arm waving activities while conducting, and upper body movements while performing, may provide them with the ideal form of exercise. Because our arms do not bear weight, we can wave them as much as we wish without damaging the joints of the elbows, and shoulders. Furthermore, the editorial writer in *Modern Medicine* reports, Dartmouth Medical School has recently shown that rowing is the best type of exercise, so far as maximal aerobic stimulation is concerned. Rowers, too, he reported, live to a very ripe old age.

Until the proof of this idea has been provided, he believes, it would be prudent for us to give it the benefit of the doubt by performing arm exercises every day and even "conducting" the music we listen to at home.

Snacks before Exercising

Taking a snack immediately before running, playing in competitive games, or other forms of heavy exercise do not help to provide extra energy, *Physician and Sportsmedicine* (12#4:89) reports. Researchers have recently shown that highly trained athletes who consumed a sweet drink or sugary snack immediately before working out on a treadmill as hard as possible performed less well and became exhausted 25 percent sooner than they did without the drink or snack.

Sugar is quickly absorbed into the bloodstream, where it stimulates the secretion of insulin that, in turn, essentially prepares the metabolism of the body for rest rather than exercise. It therefore seems advisable for athletes wishing to attain their peak performances not to snack before competing, particularly when the activity is going to be strenuous and long sustained.

Warming up Before Stretching Exercise

Stretching is important for athletes since it improves muscle flexibility and helps to prevent injury to their ligaments and joints. Thus, with exercises that stretch our hamstrings, *Physician and Sportsmedicine* (14#3:45) reports, we may protect our knees and hips from injury.

Stretching, however, will not protect us against the possibility of straining or tearing a muscle and can do harm if not performed correctly.

To do it properly and avoid injuring ourselves, stretching should never be started until we have warmed up with other exercises sufficiently to bring on sweating. In this way, our muscles get toned up before stretching begins and can better protect our joints and ligaments from becoming overstretched.

Heat or Ice for Sprains?

Standard advice about sprains has been to treat them with rest, elevation, and ice packs for the first few hours and thereafter to keep the part tightly bound.

These measures limit swelling and help to stop any further bleeding, which might cause additional damage to the injured tissues. Then, after 48 hours, it has been customary to employ hot soaks, with the thought that they help to increase the blood flow, which carries away debris.

Research, however, has demonstrated that cold is much more effective than heat during the later phase of treatment, the *Journal of the American Medical Association* (257:3132) reports. Because it penetrates more easily, cold applied on the third day of treatment induces a greater flow of blood in the deep tissue around the joint. Cold, therefore, in the form of ice packs or immersion in cold water, is now being recommended for all stages in the treatment of sprains.

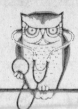

DR. ALEXANDER GRANT'S
HEALTH GAZETTE™
A DIGEST OF MEDICAL FACTS AND NEWS
PUBLISHED AS **HEALTHWISE** FROM MAY 1978 THRU JULY 1988